This book

Belongs to

....

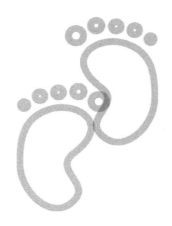

My Pregnancy Journey

Photograph Paste here

1 Week

_____

_____

_____

_____

Photograph Paste here

2 Week

_____

_____

_____

_____

My Pregnancy Journey

<table>
<tr><td>Photograph Paste here</td><td>3 Week</td></tr>
</table>

Photograph
Paste here

3 Week

_____
_____
_____
_____
_____

Photograph
Paste here

4 Week

_____
_____
_____
_____
_____

My Pregnancy Journey

5 Week

Photograph
Paste here

_____

_____

_____

_____

6 Week

Photograph
Paste here

_____

_____

_____

_____

My Pregnancy Journey

7 Week

Photograph
Paste here

_____

_____

_____

_____

8 Week

Photograph
Paste here

_____

_____

_____

_____

My Pregnancy Journey

9 Week

Photograph
Paste here

_____
_____
_____
_____

10 Week

Photograph
Paste here

_____
_____
_____
_____

My Pregnancy Journey

Photograph Paste here

11 Week

_____

_____

_____

_____

Photograph Paste here

12 Week

_____

_____

_____

_____

My Pregnancy Journey

13 Week

Photograph
Paste here

_____

_____

_____

_____

14 Week

Photograph
Paste here

_____

_____

_____

_____

My Pregnancy Journey

15 Week

Photograph
Paste here

_____

_____

_____

_____

16 Week

Photograph
Paste here

_____

_____

_____

_____

My Pregnancy Journey

17 Week

Photograph
Paste here

_____

_____

_____

_____

18 Week

Photograph
Paste here

_____

_____

_____

_____

My Pregnancy Journey

Photograph Paste here

19 Week

_____

_____

_____

_____

_____

Photograph Paste here

20 Week

_____

_____

_____

_____

_____

My Pregnancy Journey

21 Week

Photograph
Paste here

_____

_____

_____

_____

22 Week

Photograph
Paste here

_____

_____

_____

_____

My Pregnancy Journey

23 Week

Photograph
Paste here

_____

_____

_____

_____

24 Week

Photograph
Paste here

_____

_____

_____

_____

My Pregnancy Journey

25 Week

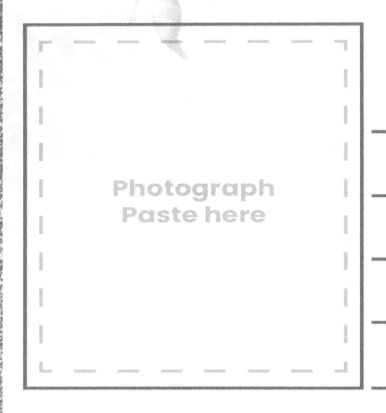

Photograph
Paste here

_____

_____

_____

_____

26 Week

Photograph
Paste here

_____

_____

_____

_____

My Pregnancy Journey

27 Week

Photograph
Paste here

_____
_____
_____
_____
_____

28 Week

Photograph
Paste here

_____
_____
_____
_____
_____

My Pregnancy Journey

Photograph Paste here

29 Week

_____

_____

_____

_____

Photograph Paste here

30 Week

_____

_____

_____

_____

My Pregnancy Journey

31 Week

Photograph
Paste here

_____

_____

_____

_____

32 Week

Photograph
Paste here

_____

_____

_____

_____

My Pregnancy Journey

33 Week

Photograph
Paste here

_____

_____

_____

_____

34 Week

Photograph
Paste here

_____

_____

_____

_____

My Pregnancy Journey

Photograph Paste here

35 Week

_____
_____
_____
_____

Photograph Paste here

36 Week

_____
_____
_____
_____

My Pregnancy Journey

37 Week

Photograph
Paste here

_____

_____

_____

_____

38 Week

Photograph
Paste here

_____

_____

_____

_____

My Pregnancy Journey

39 Week

Photograph
Paste here

_____

_____

_____

_____

40 Week

Photograph
Paste here

_____

_____

_____

_____

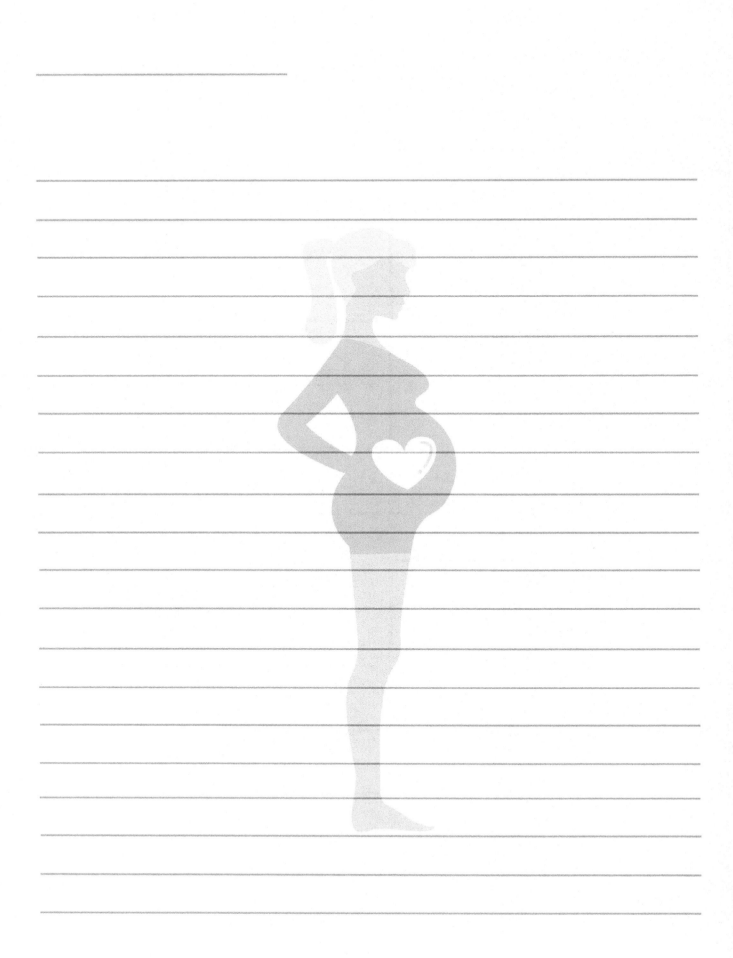

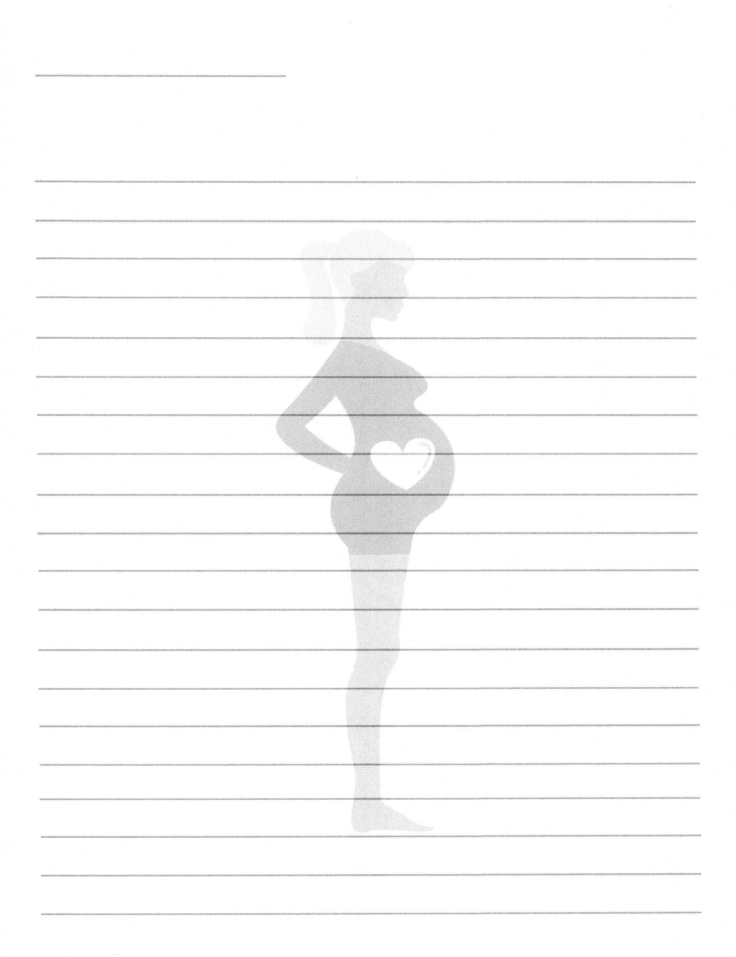

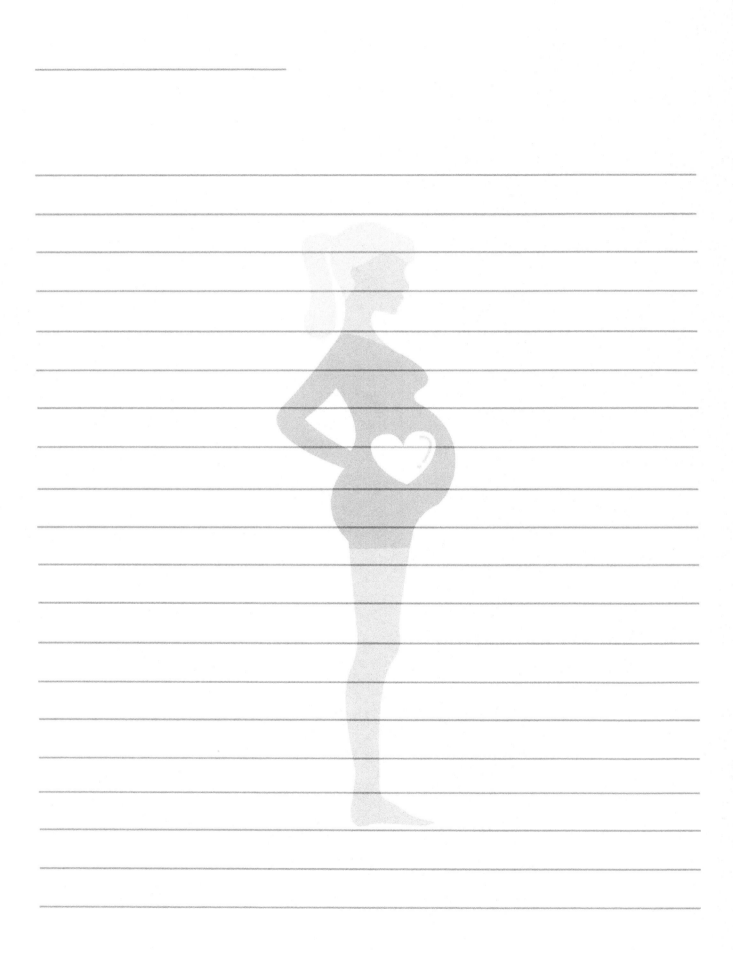

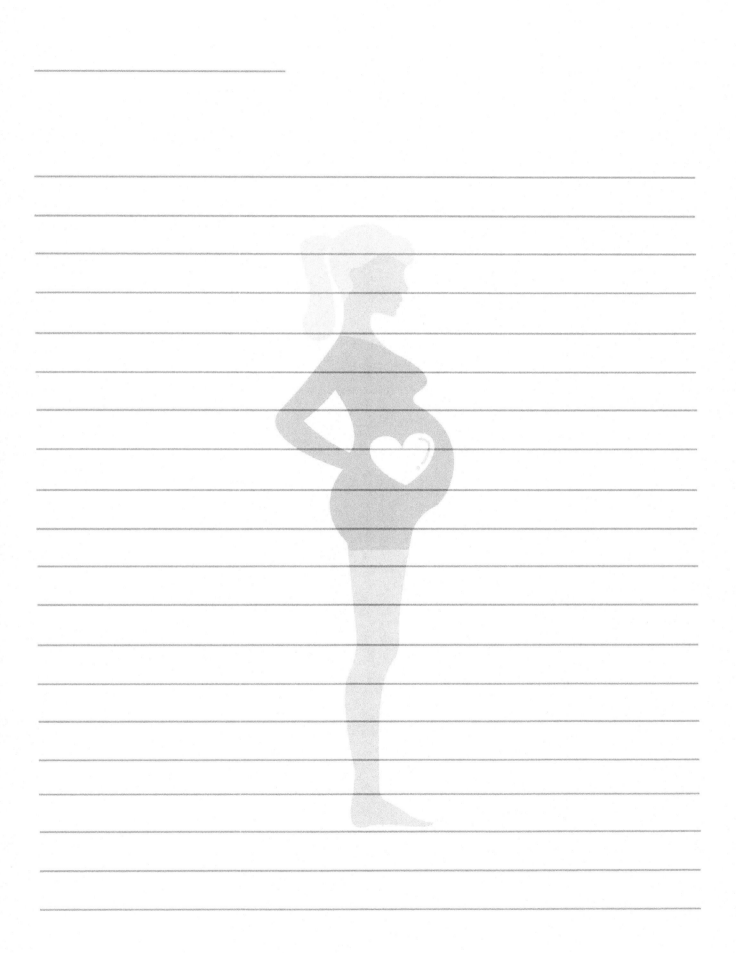

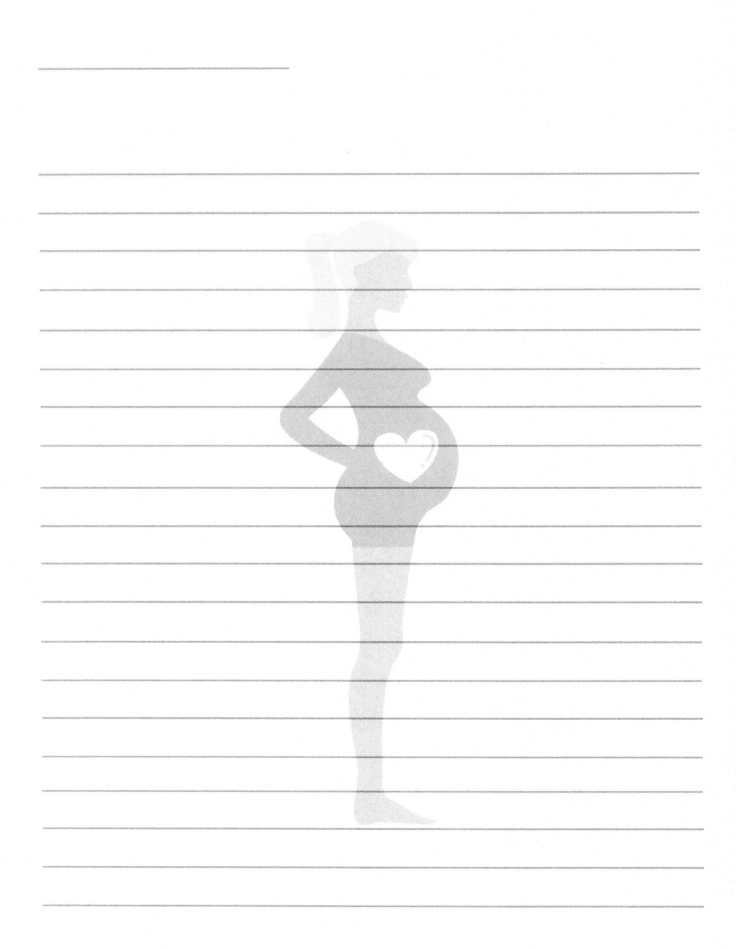

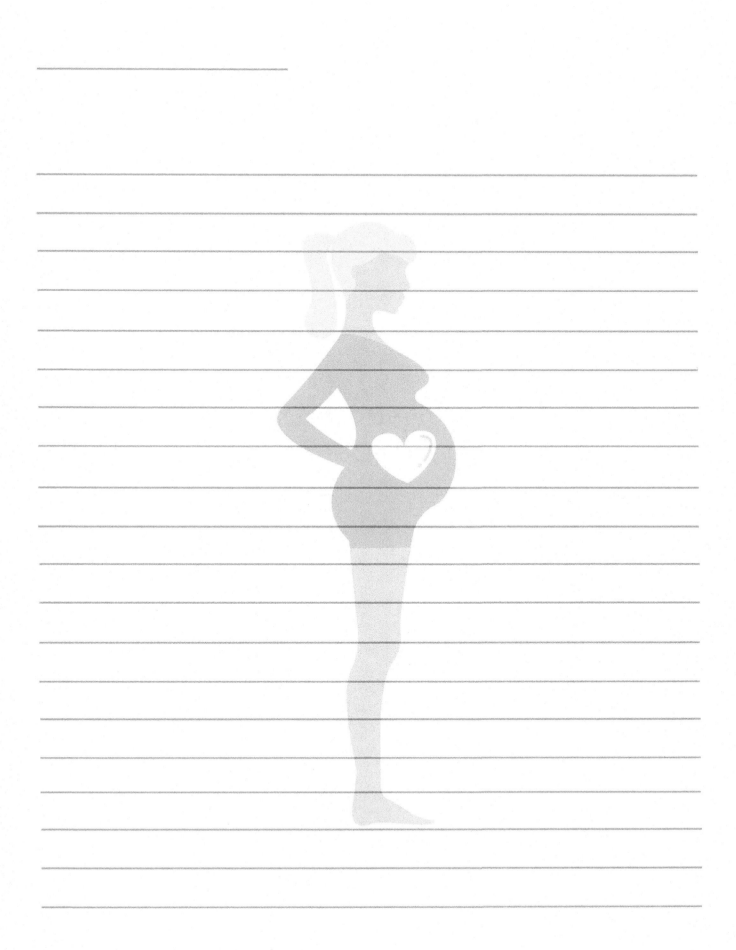

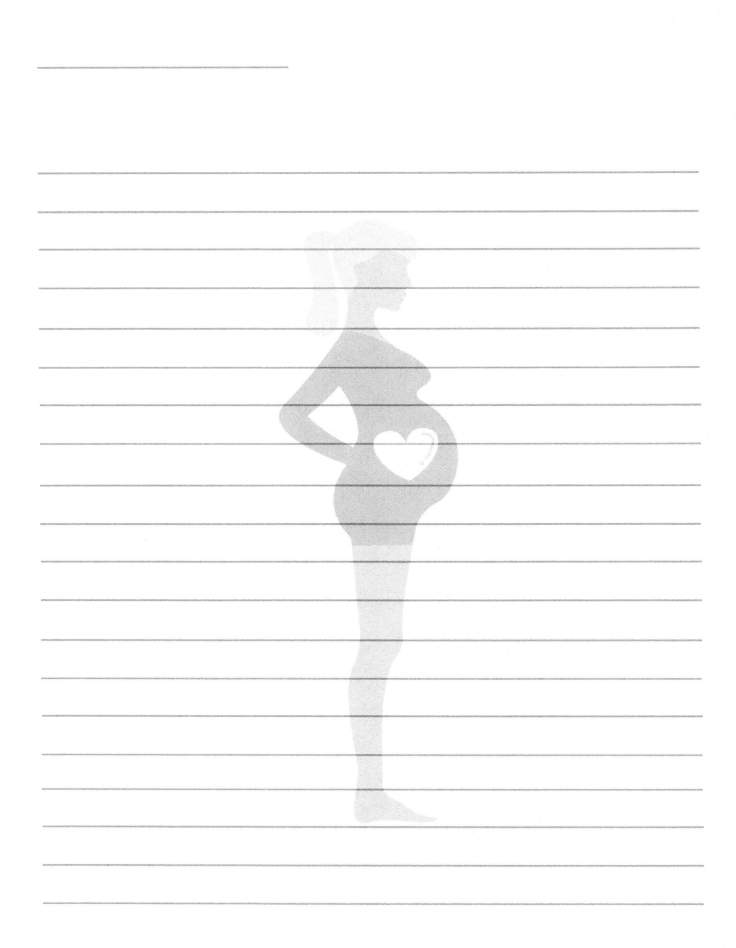

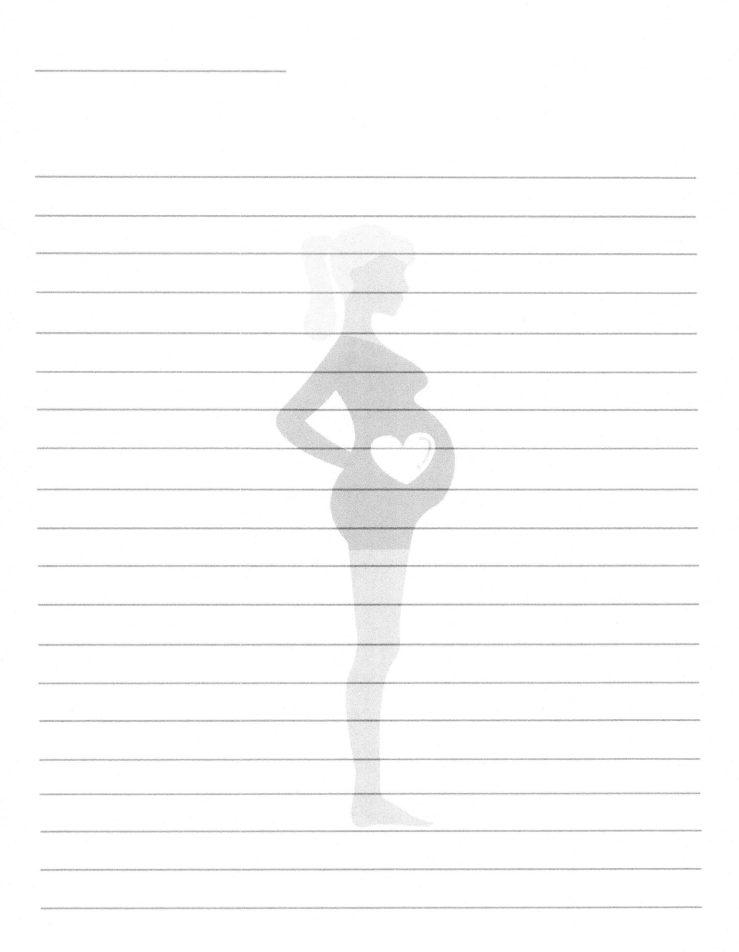

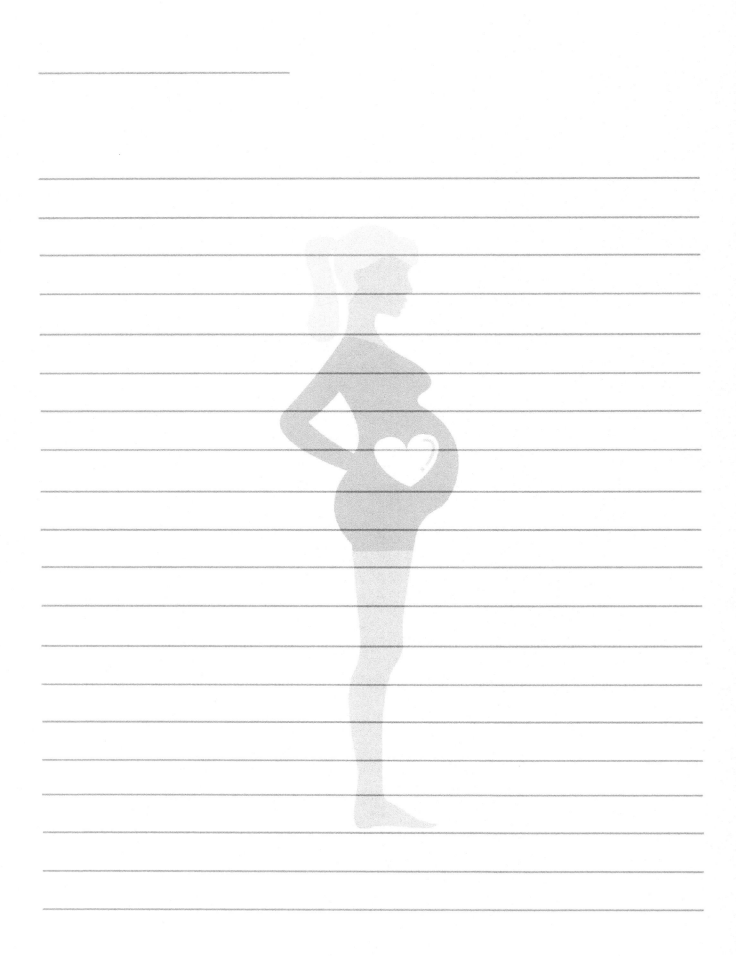

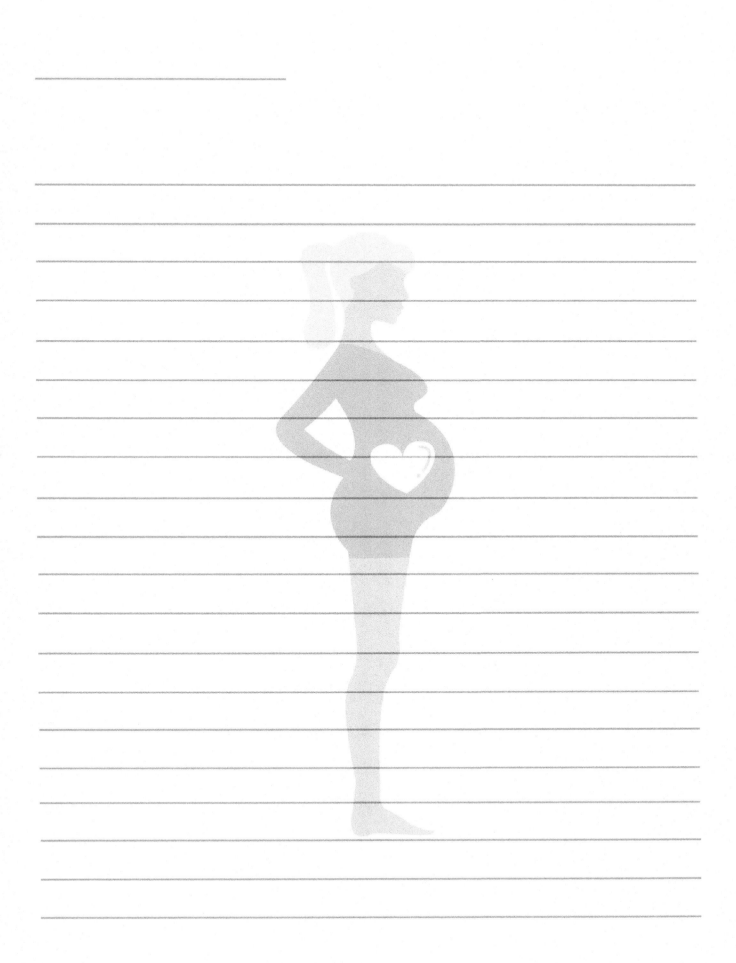

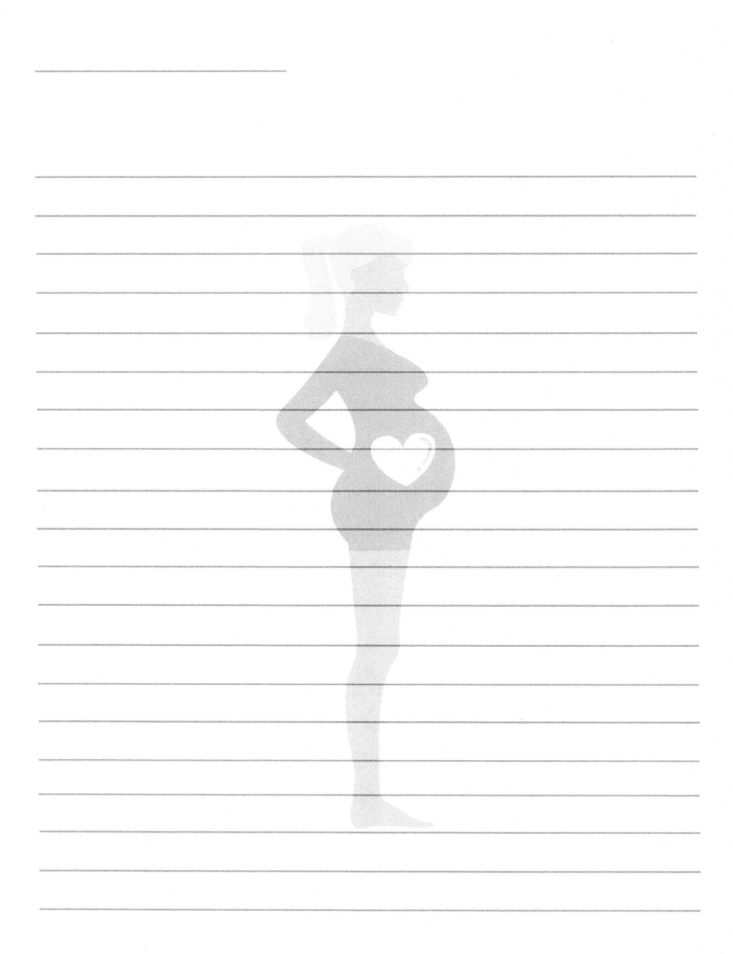

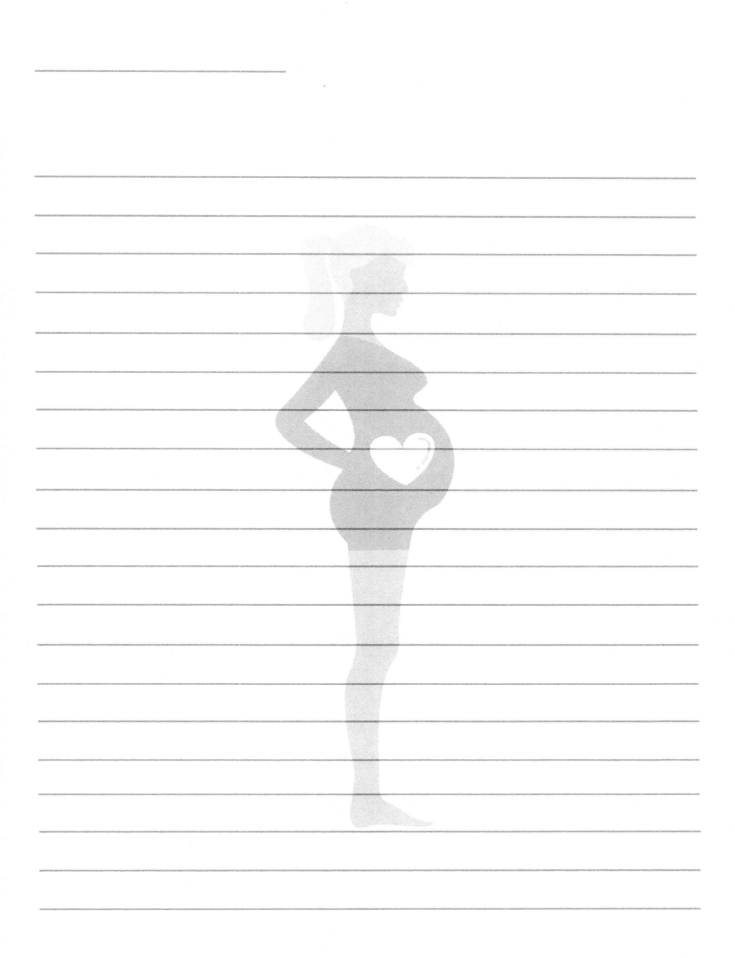

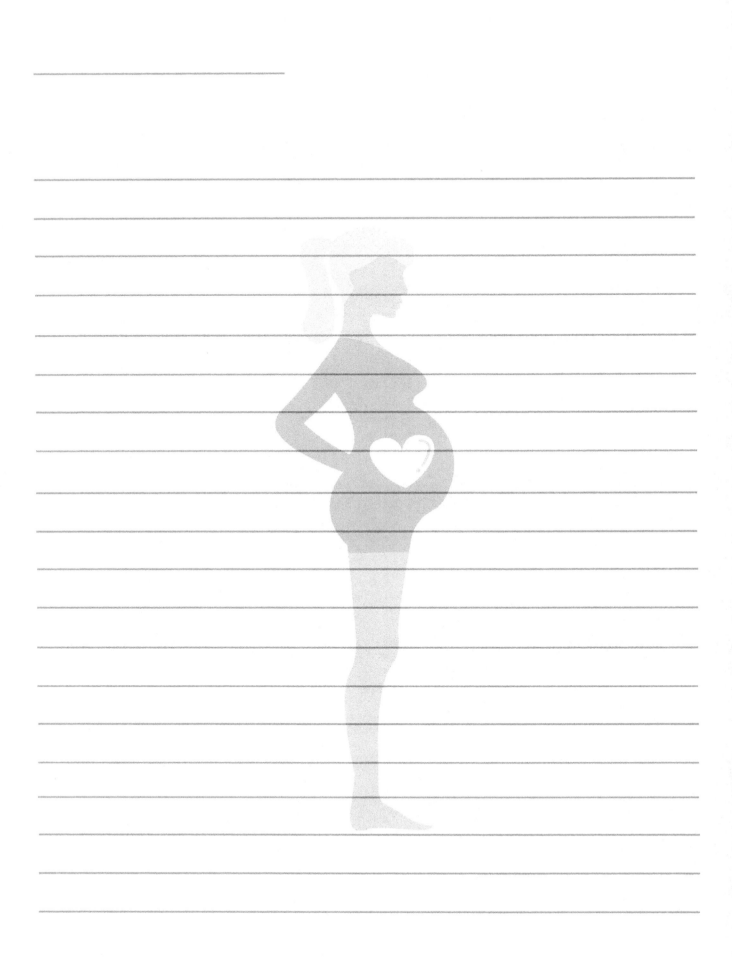

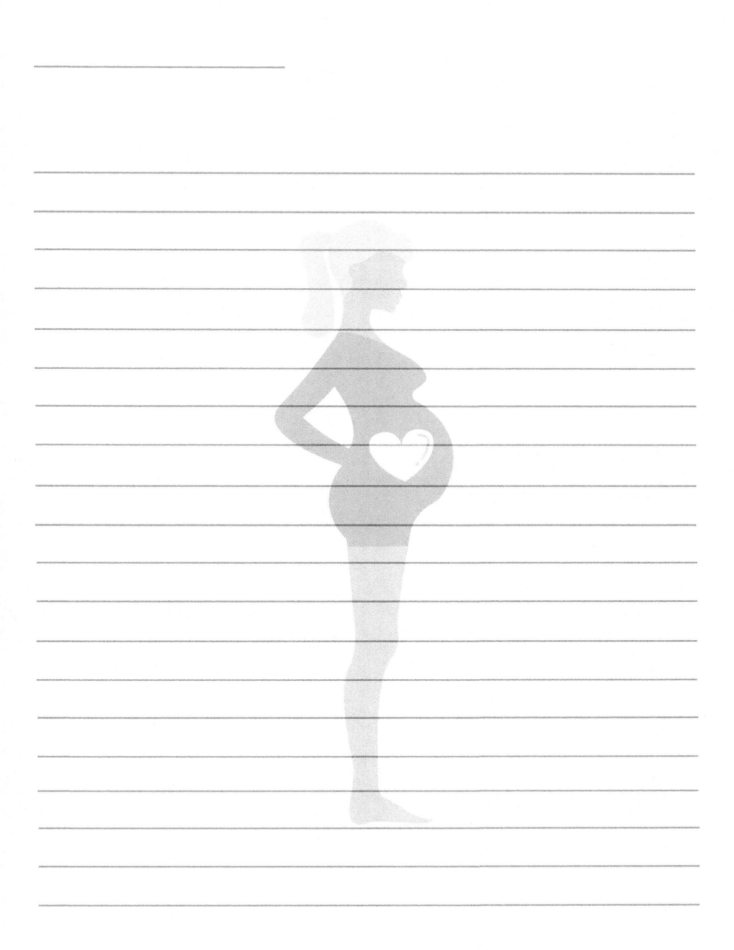

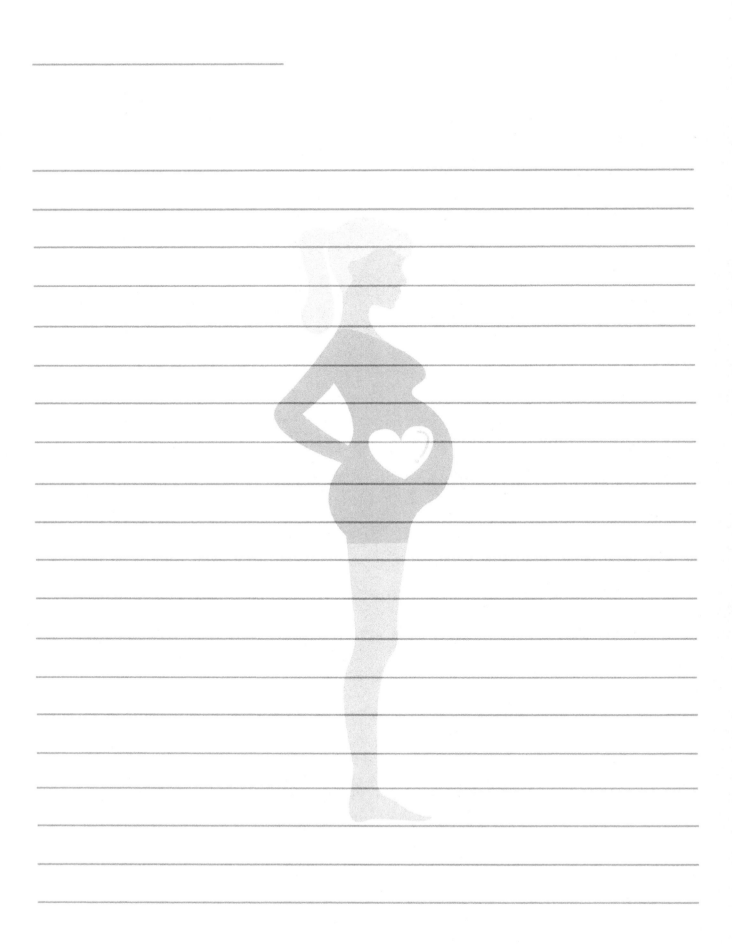

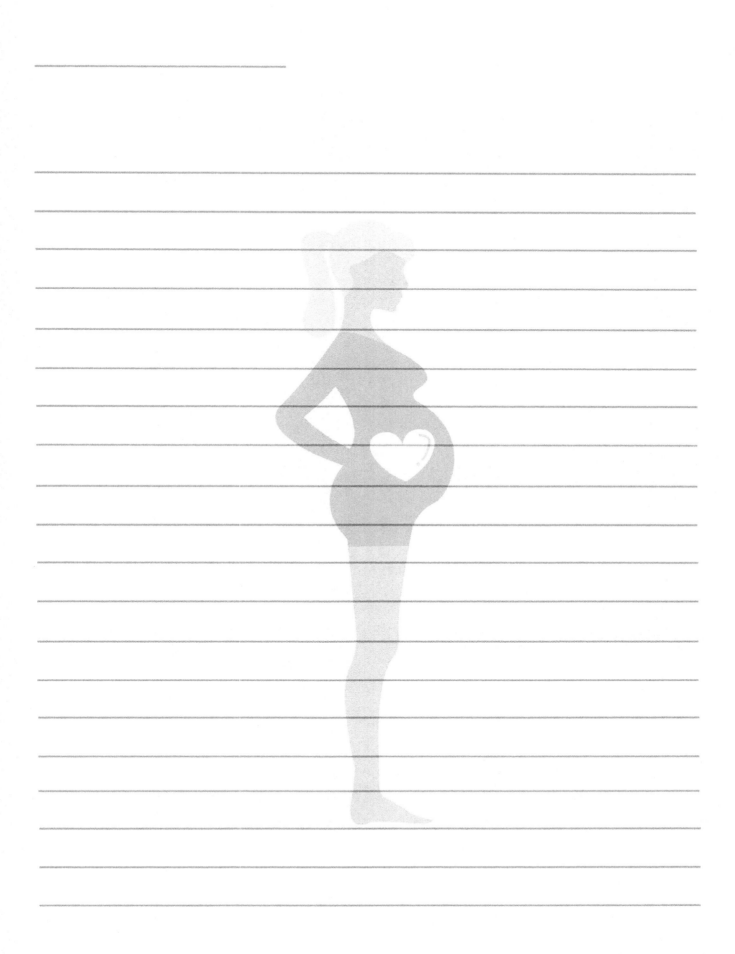

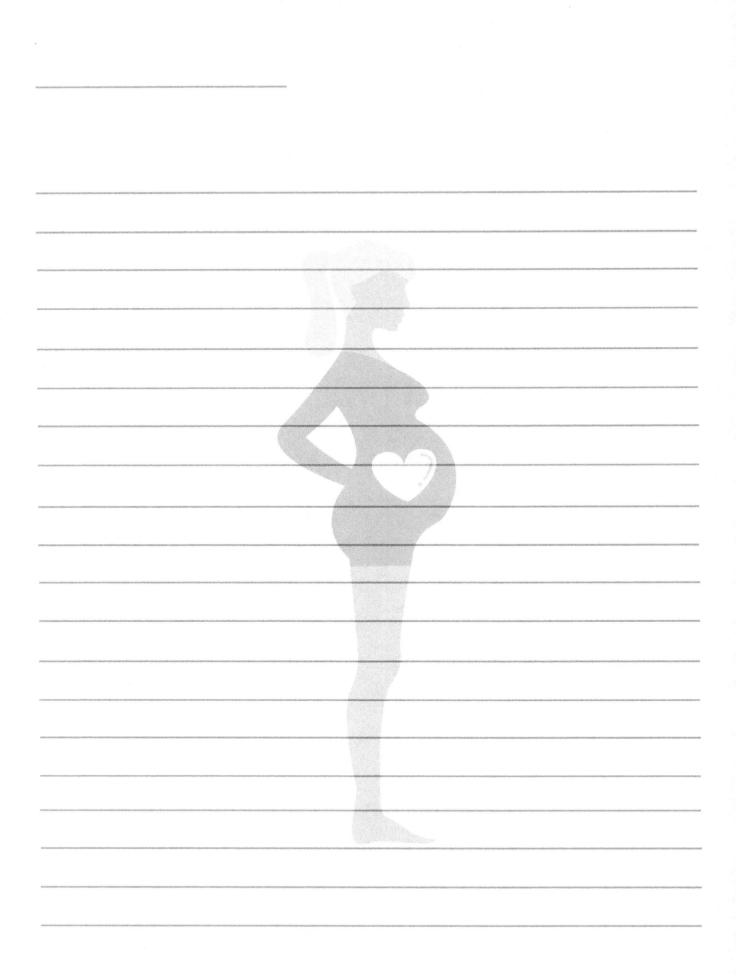

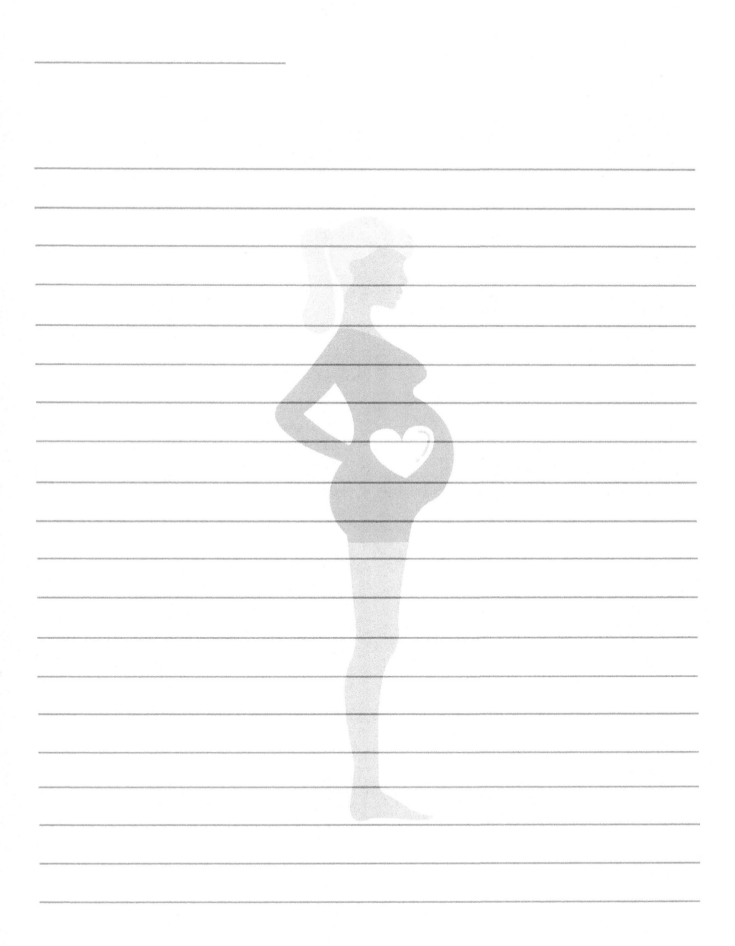

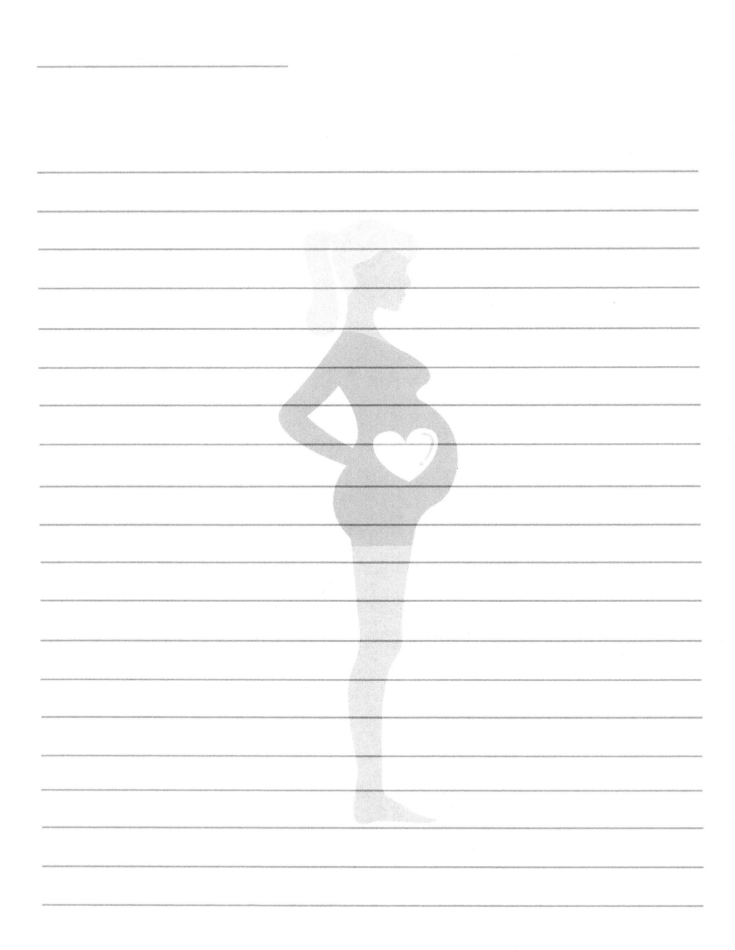

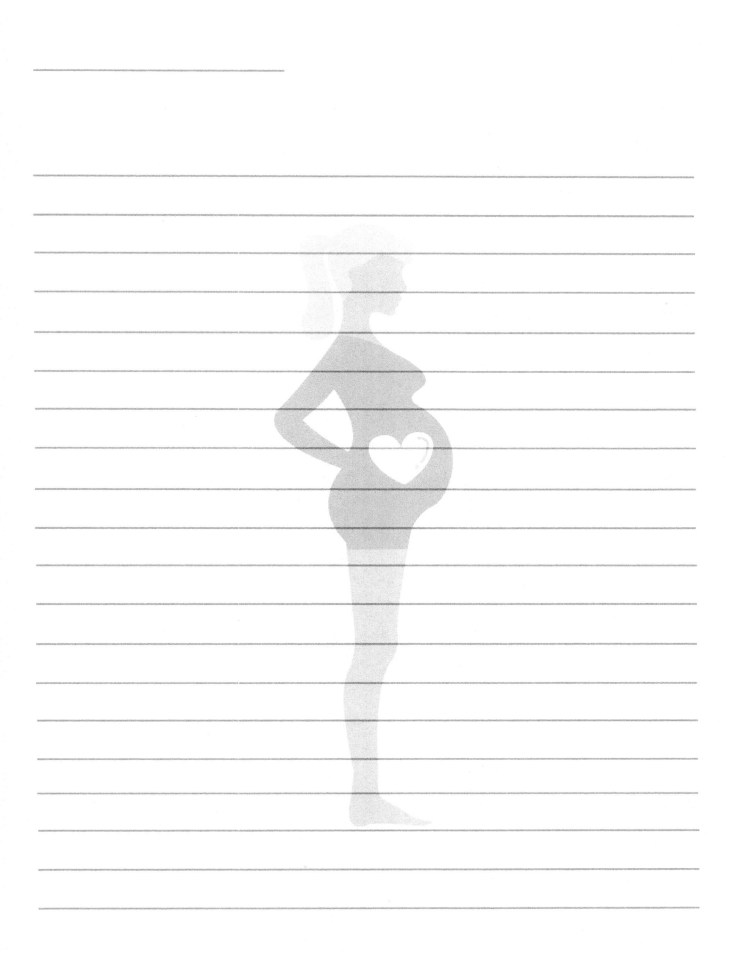

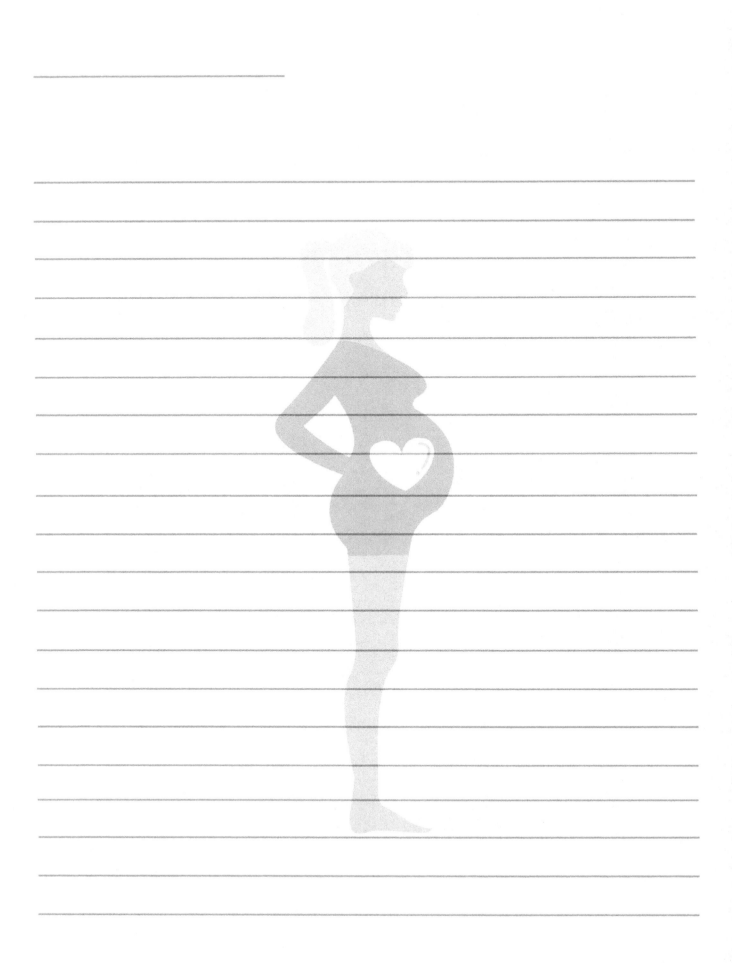

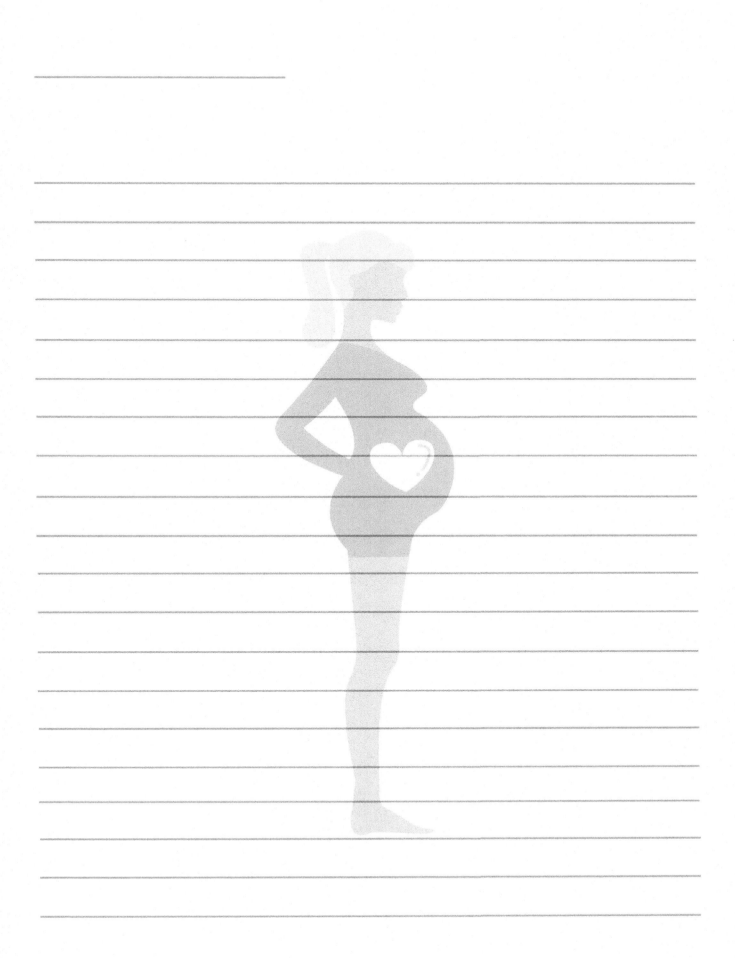

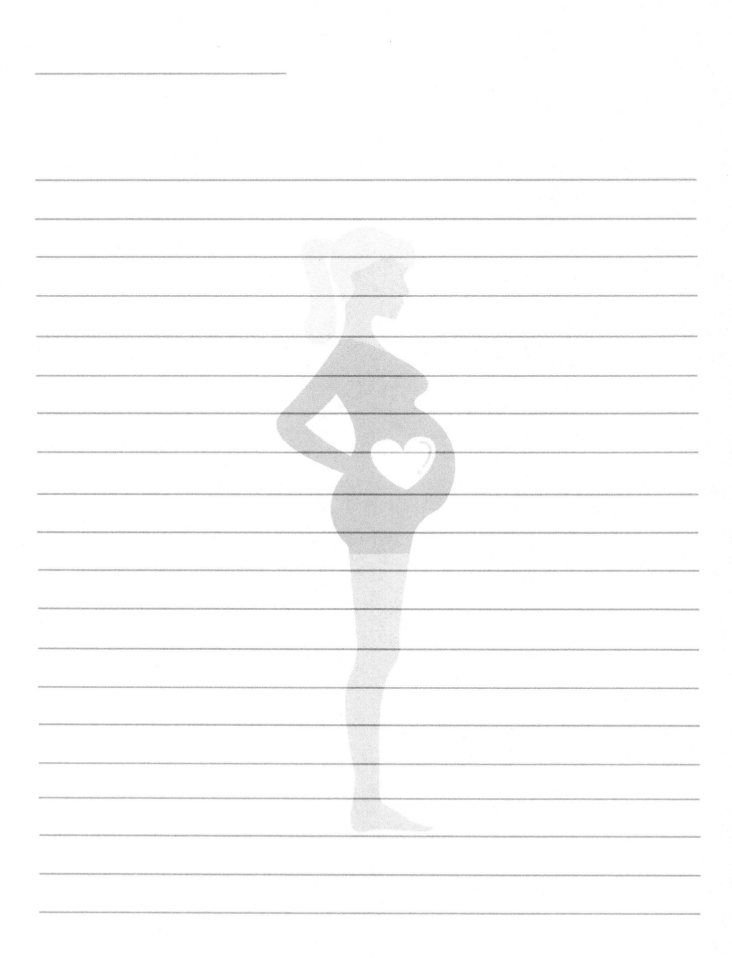

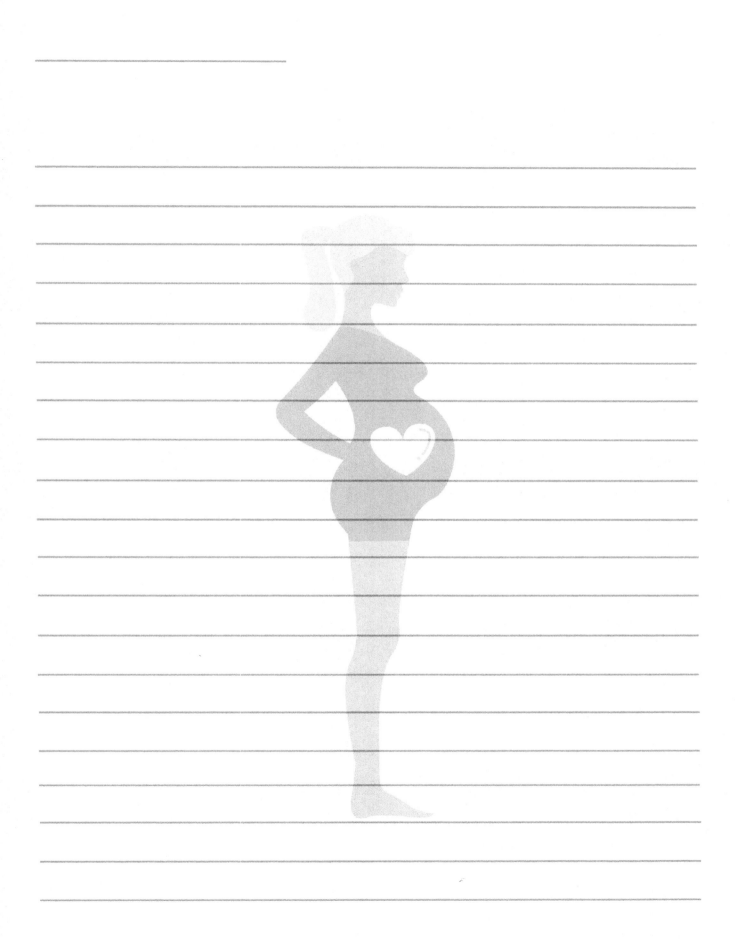

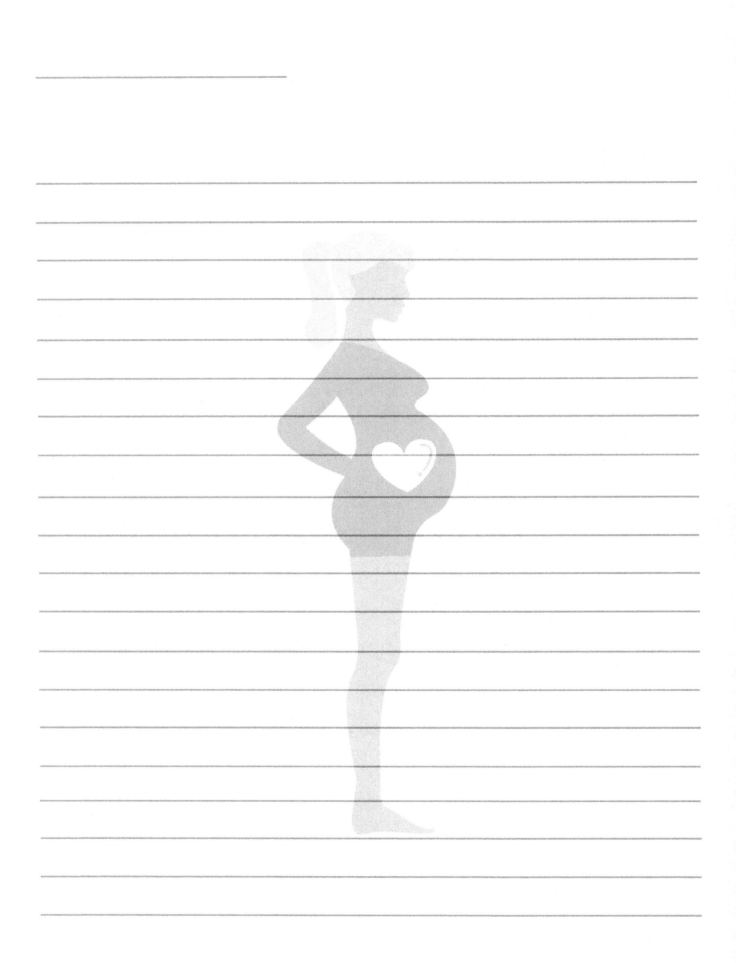

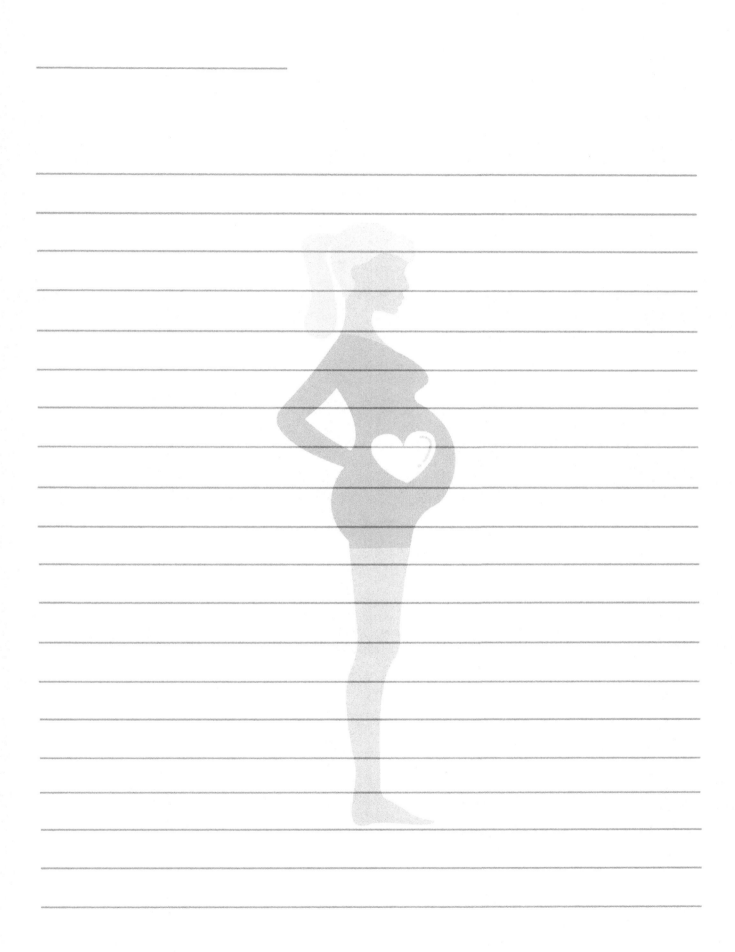

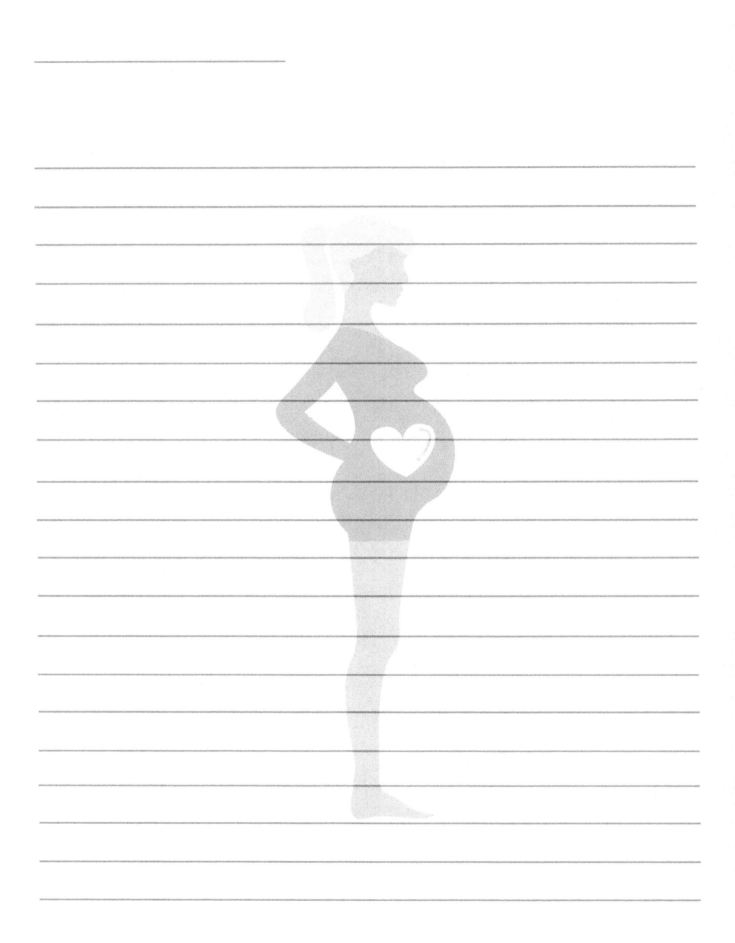

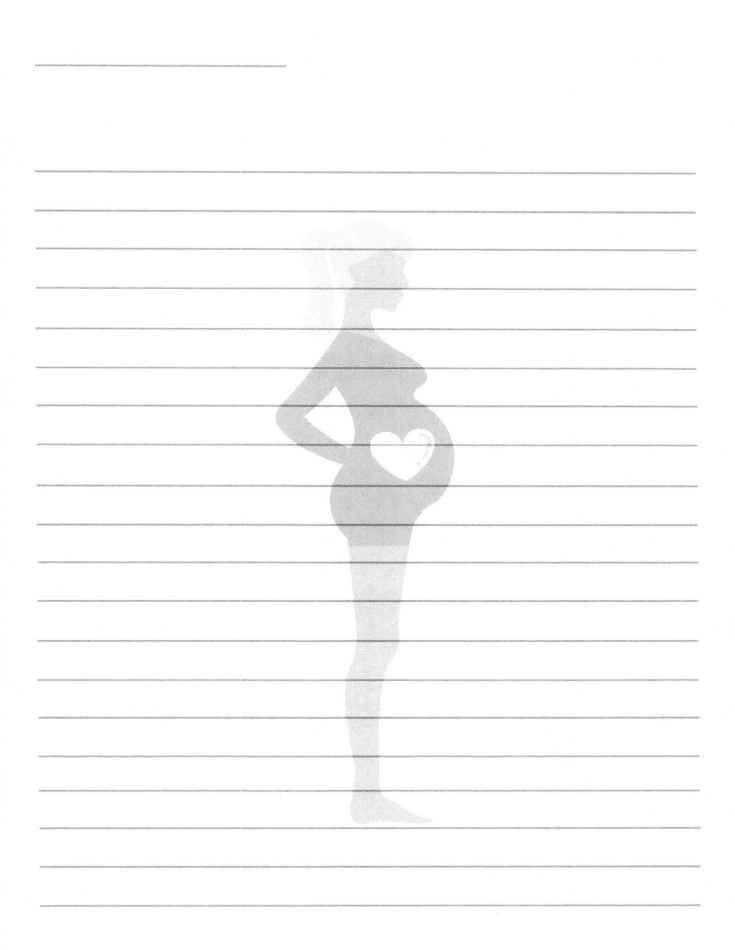

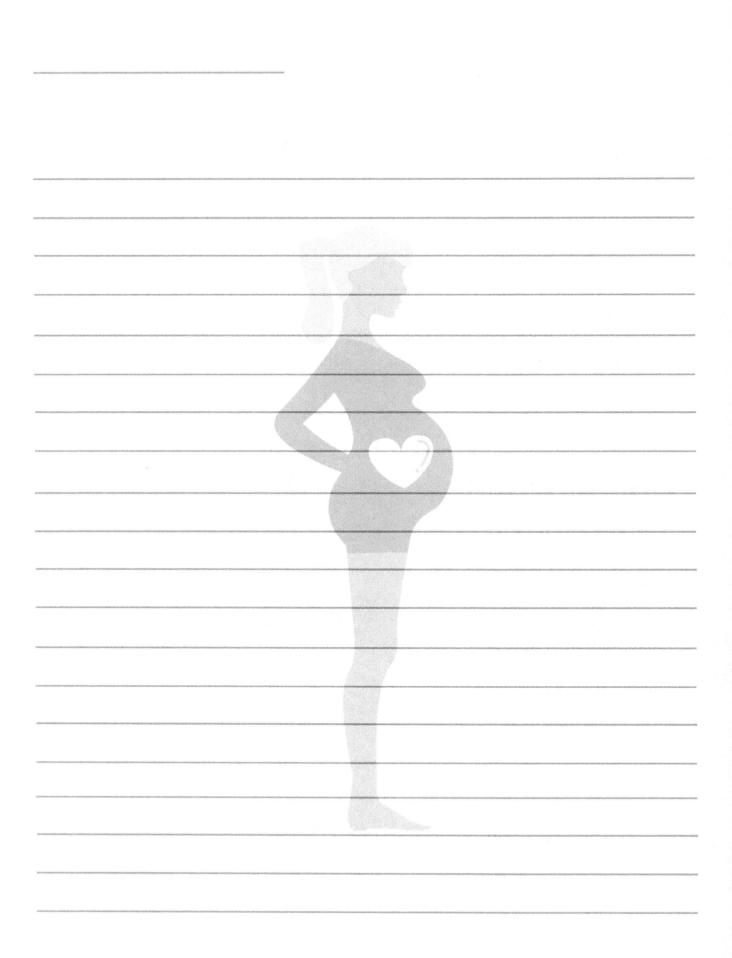

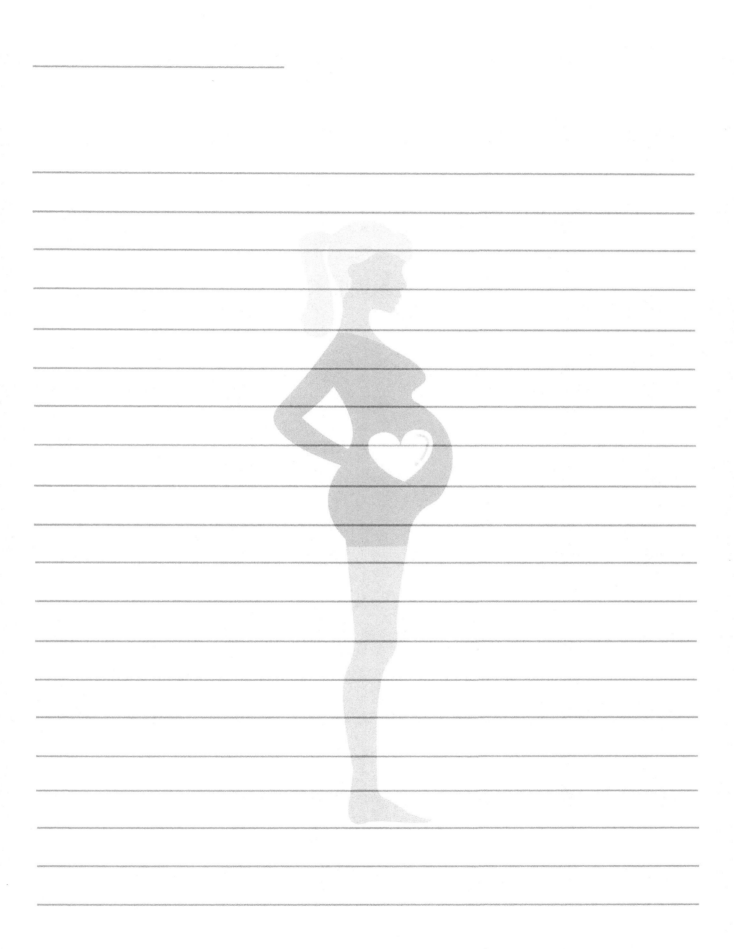

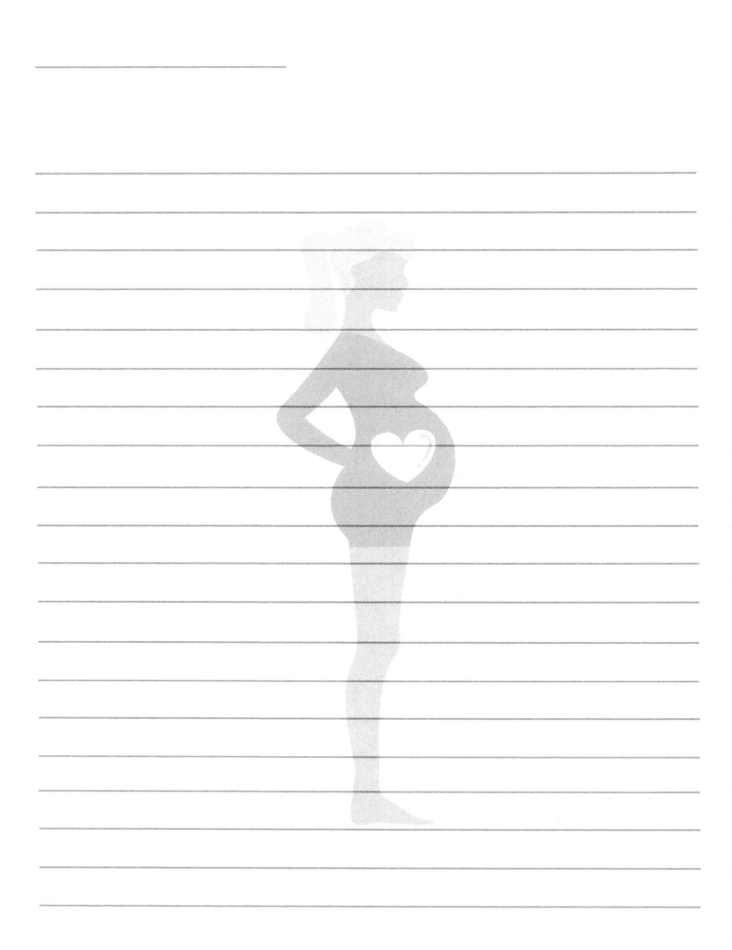

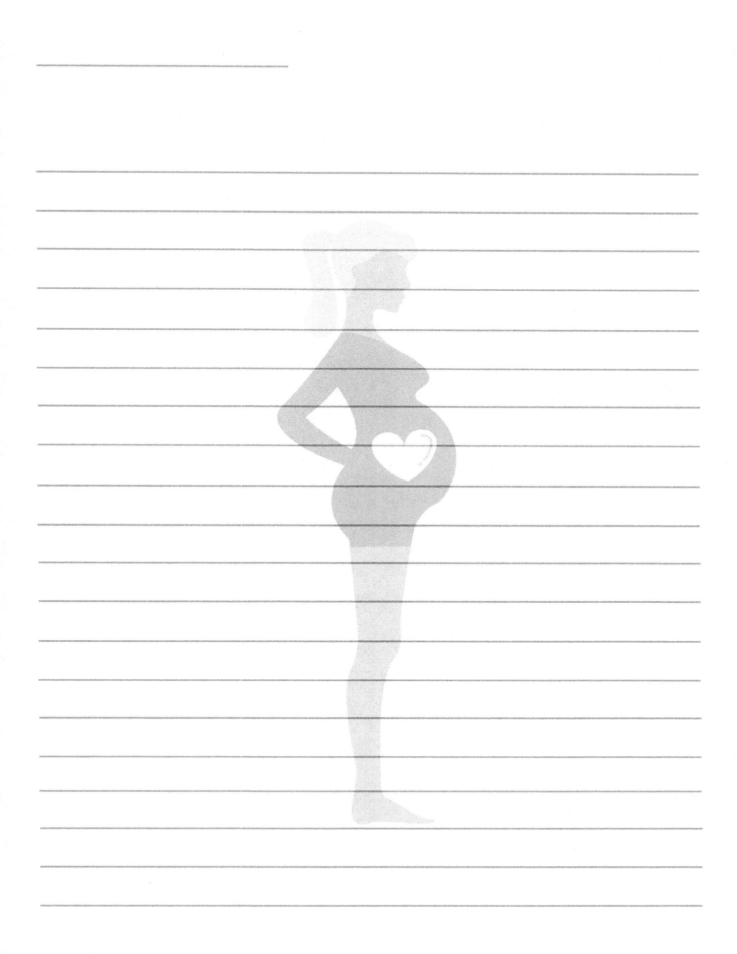

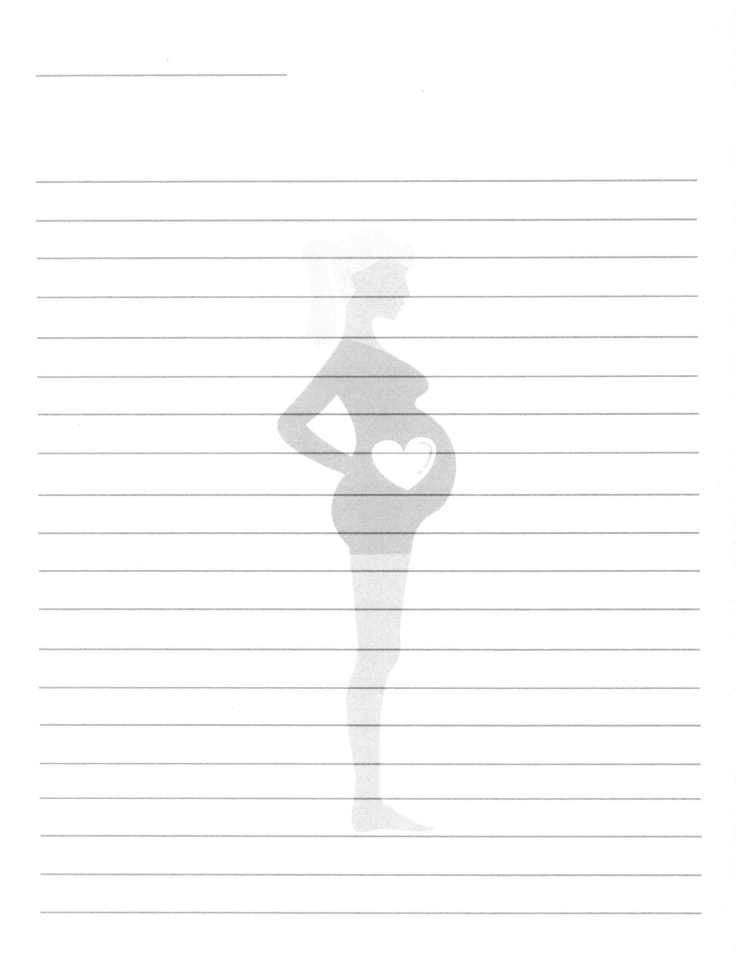

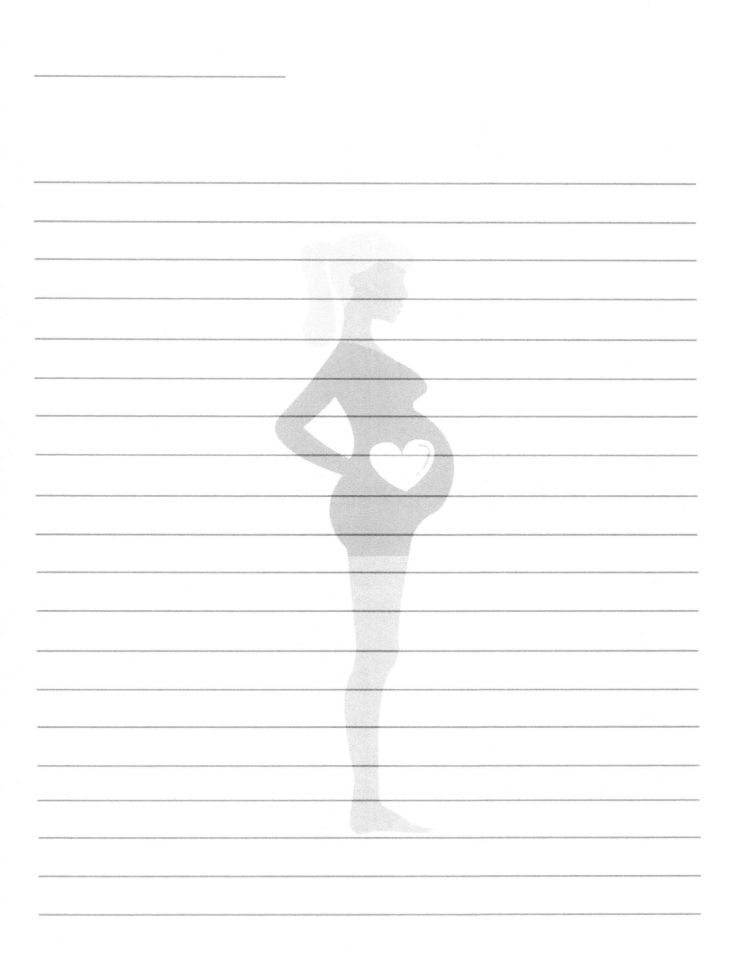

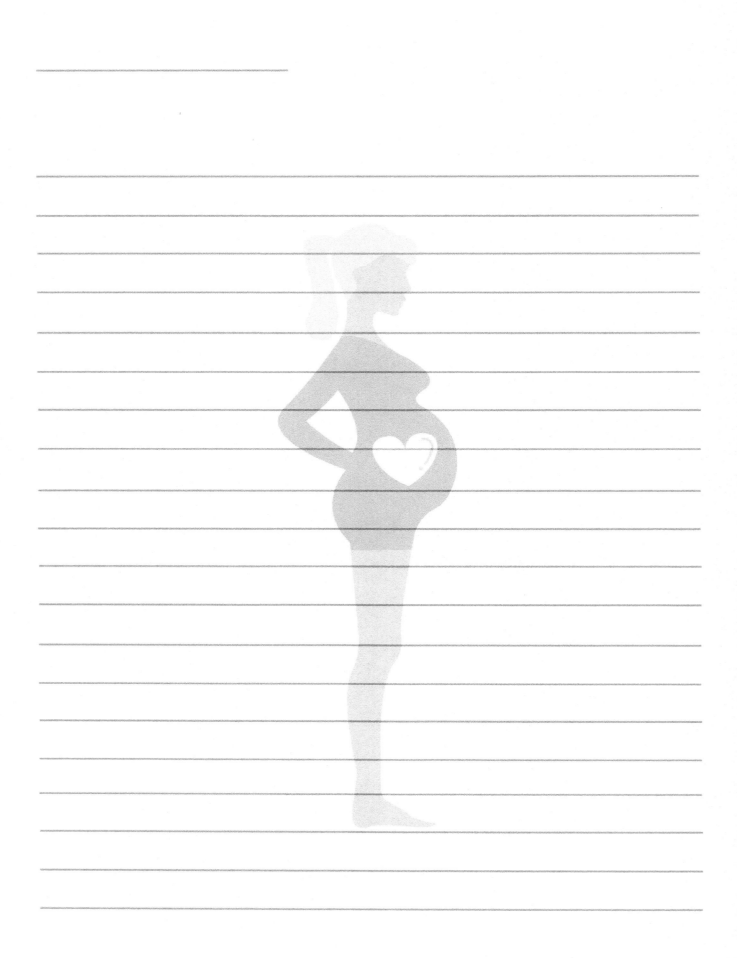

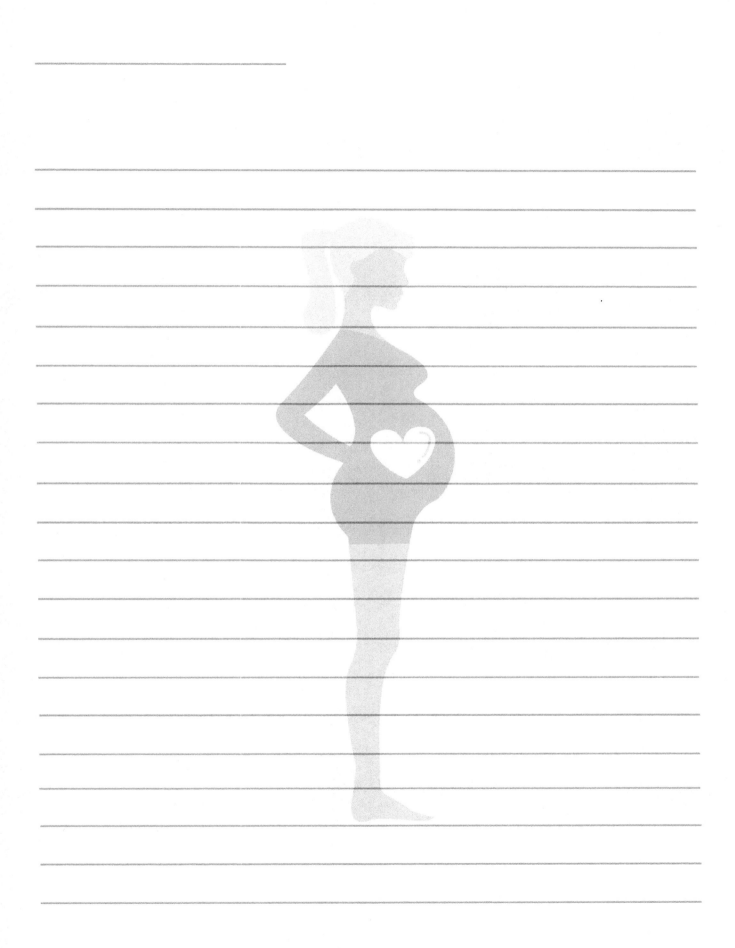

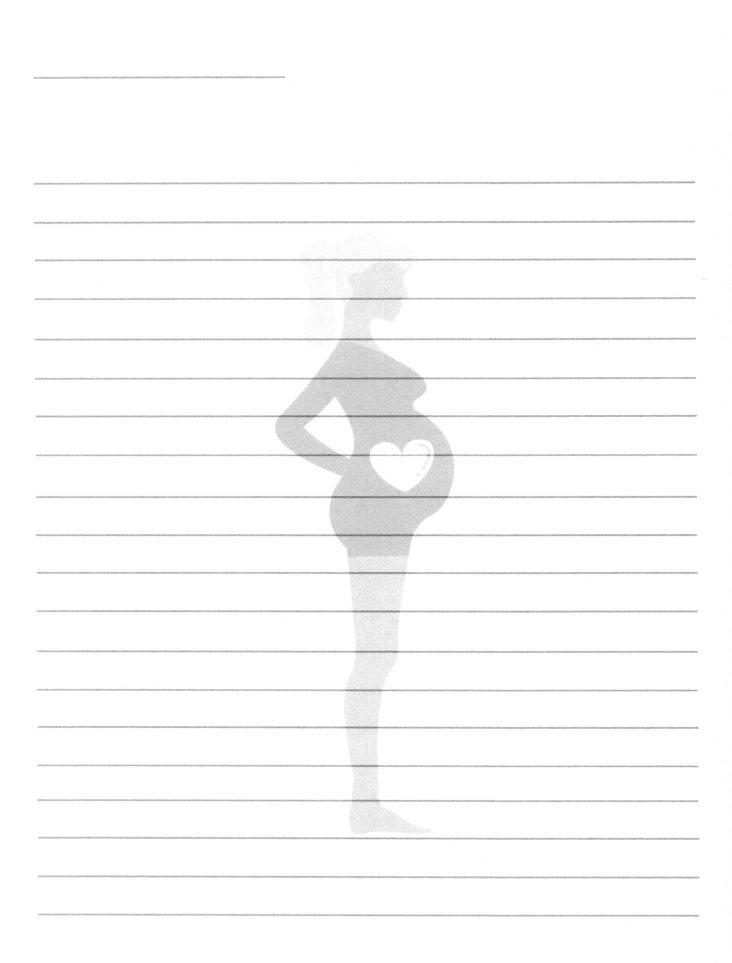

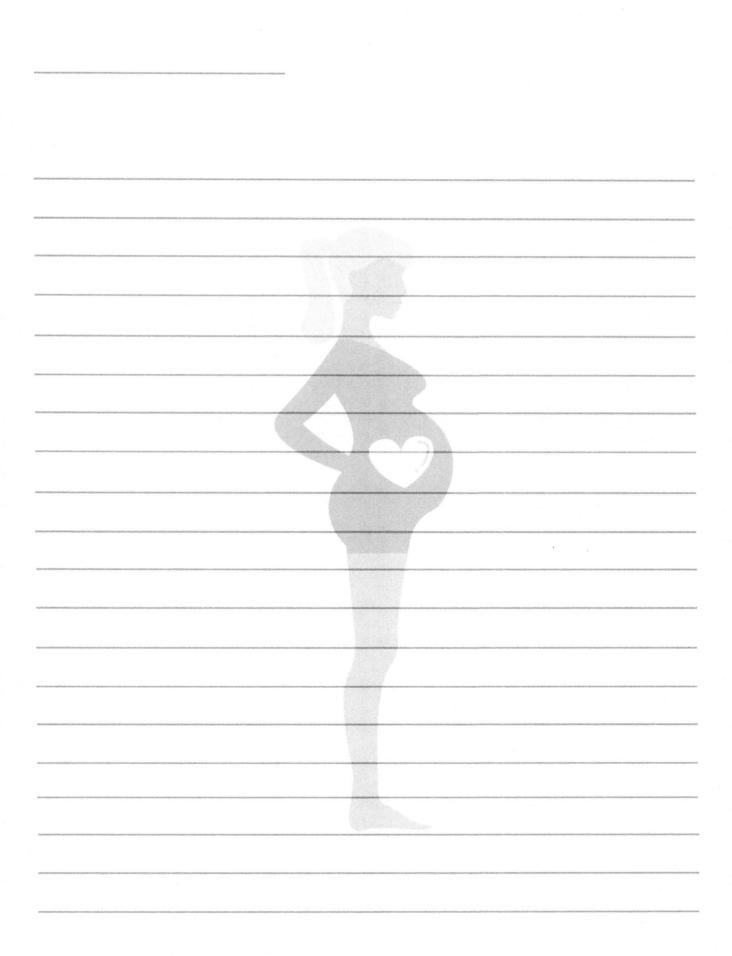

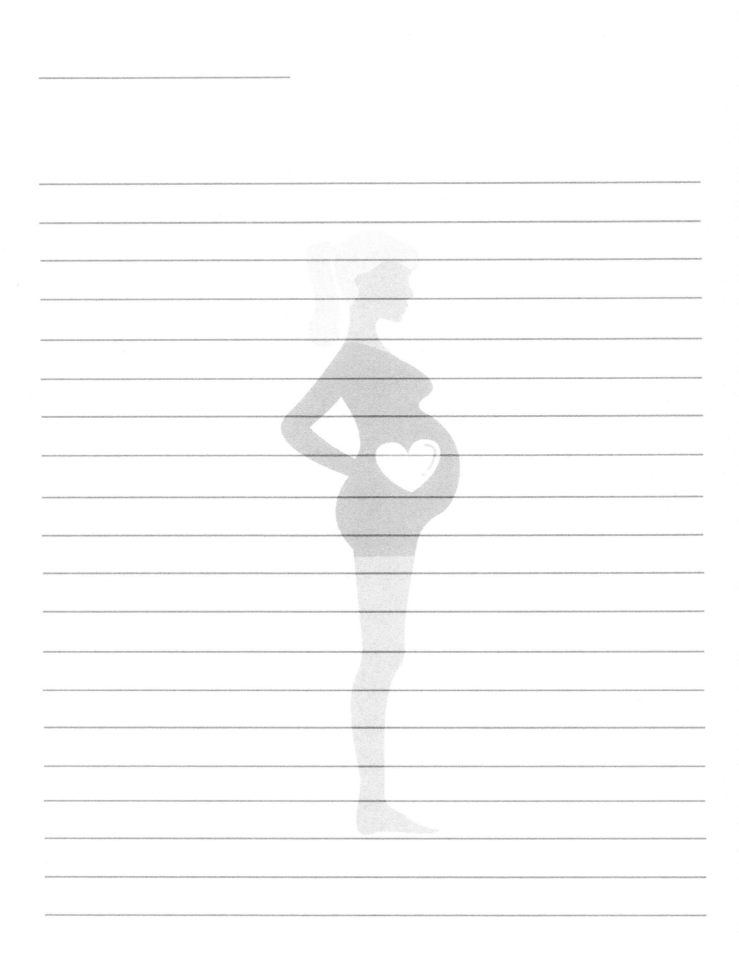

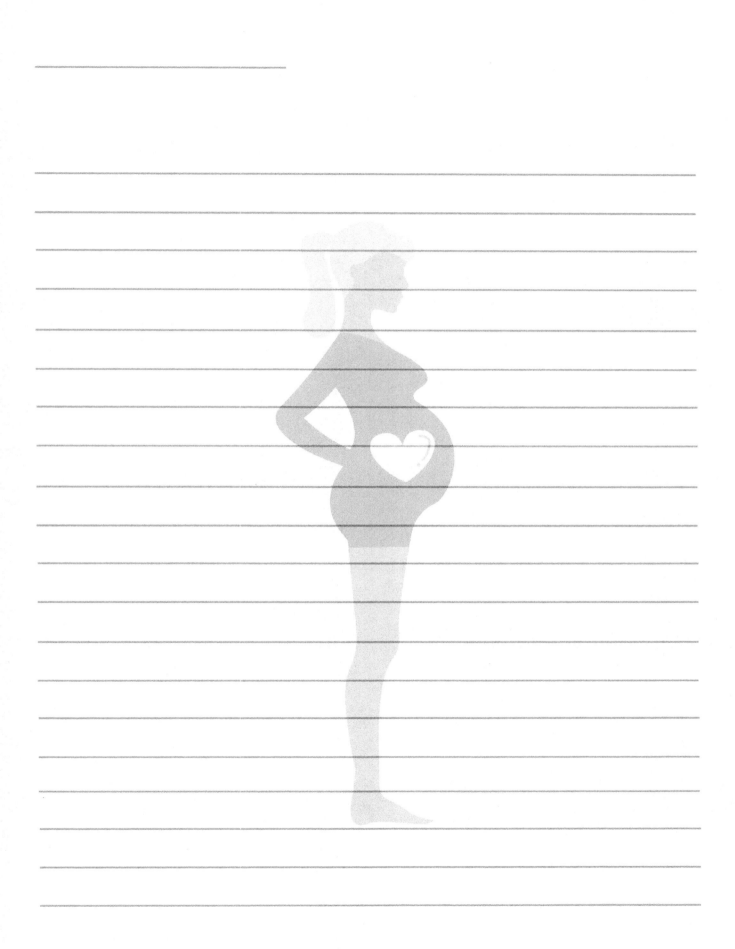

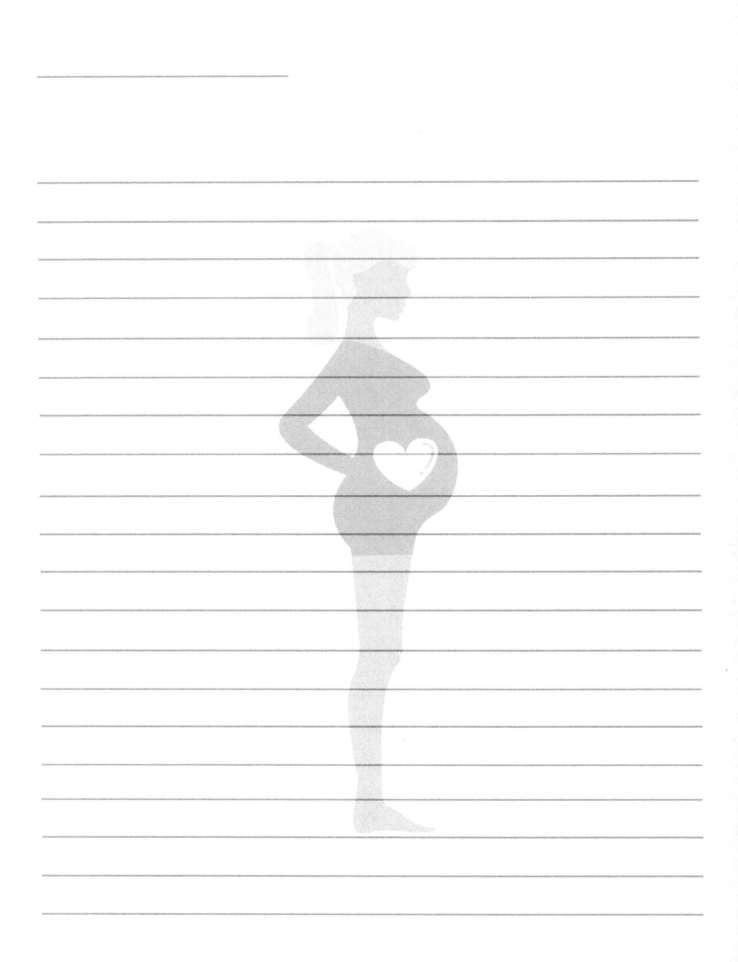

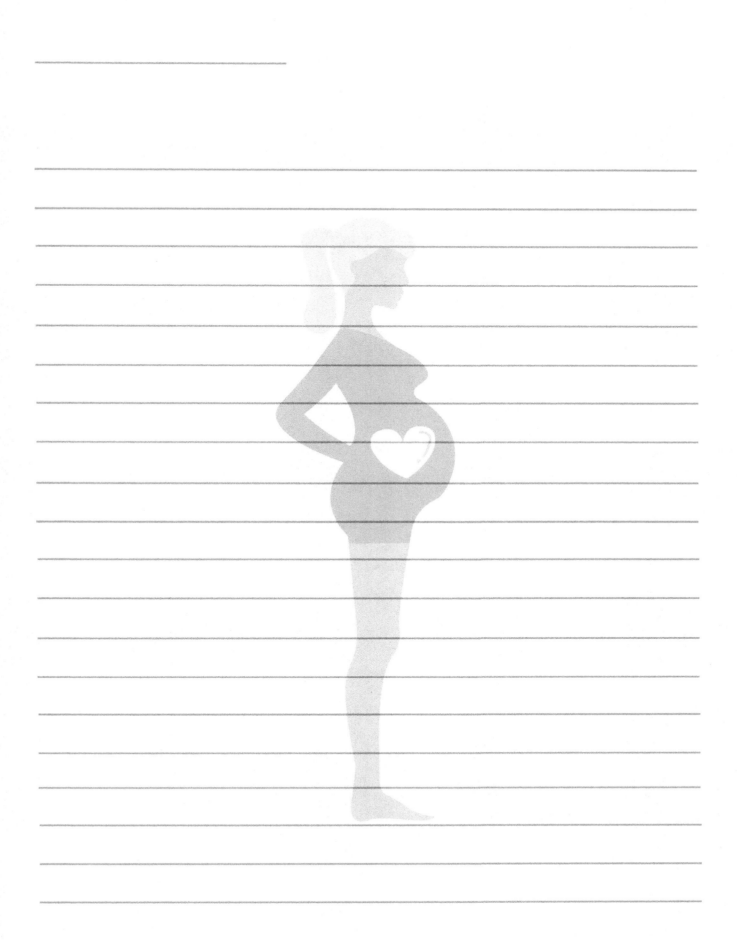

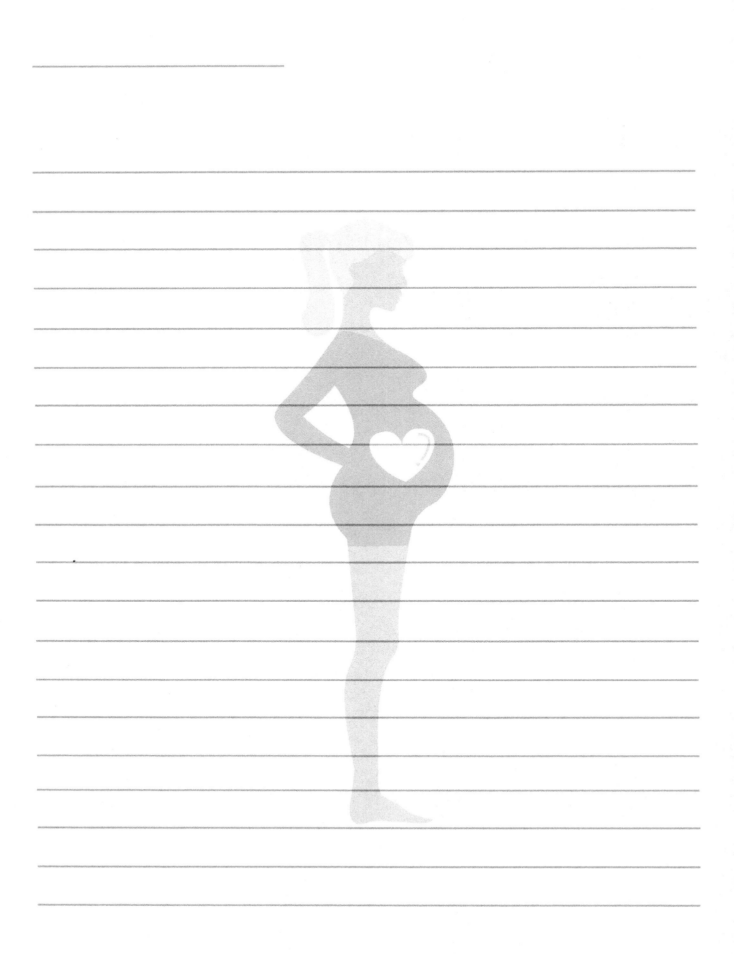

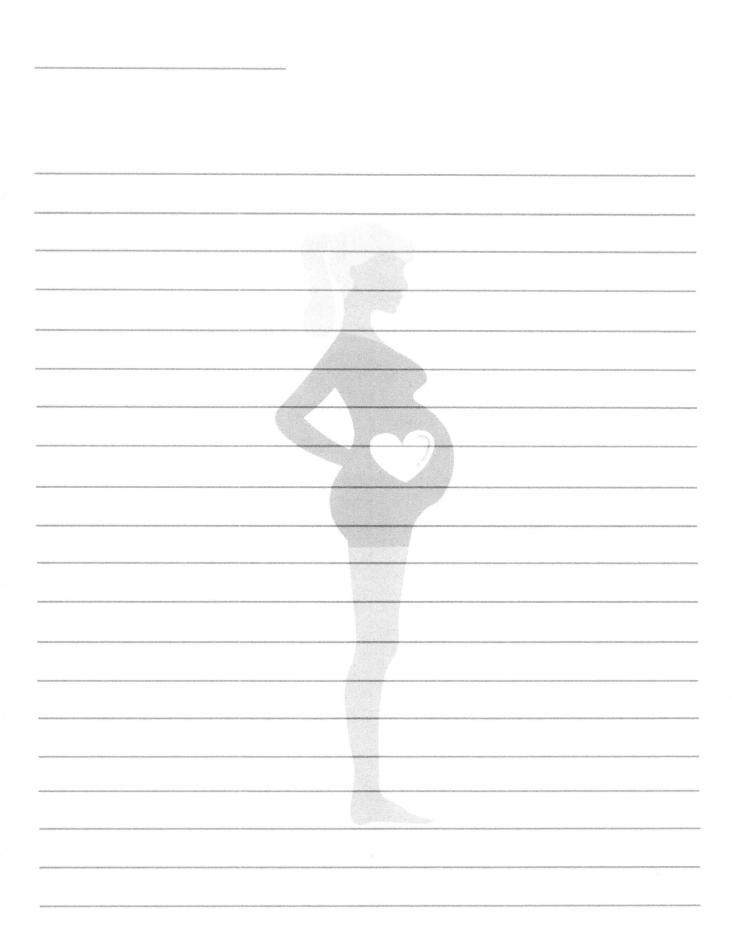

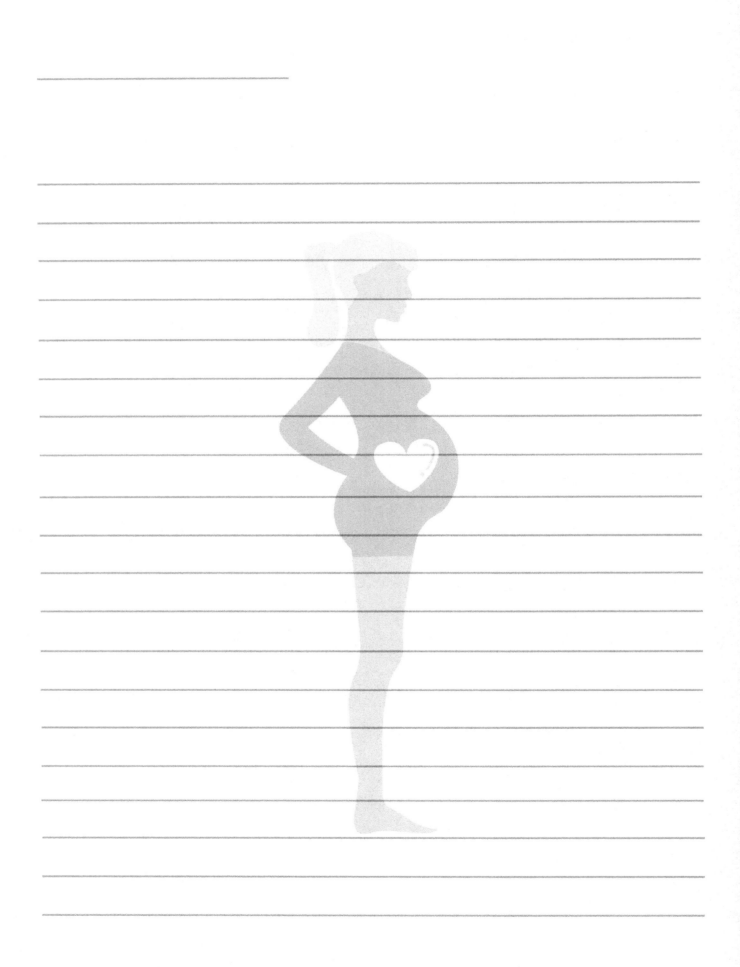

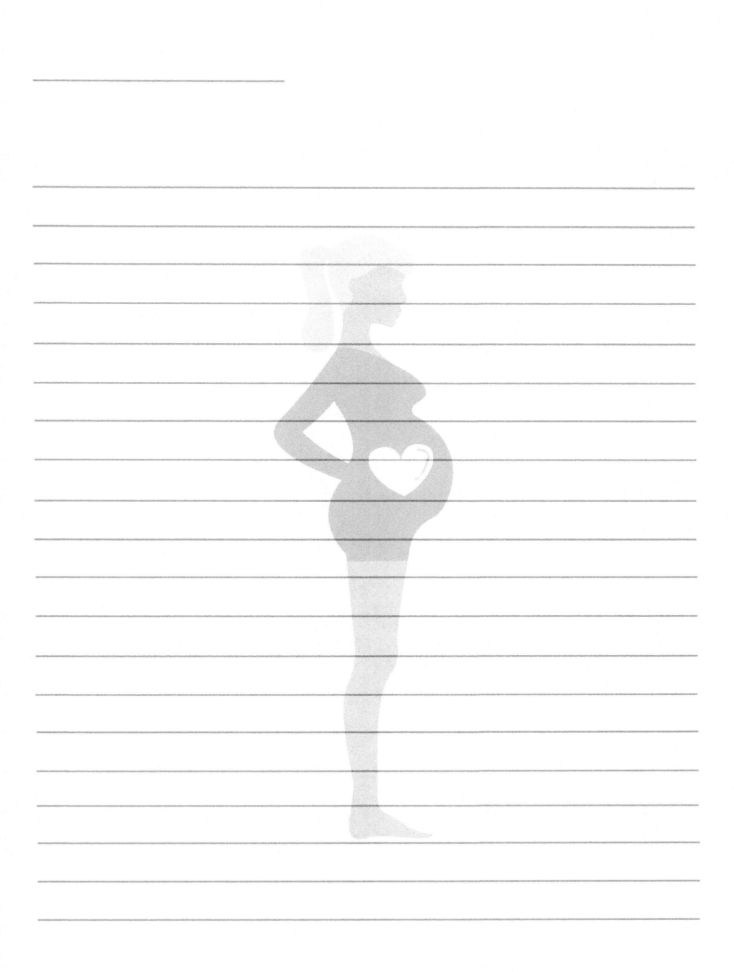

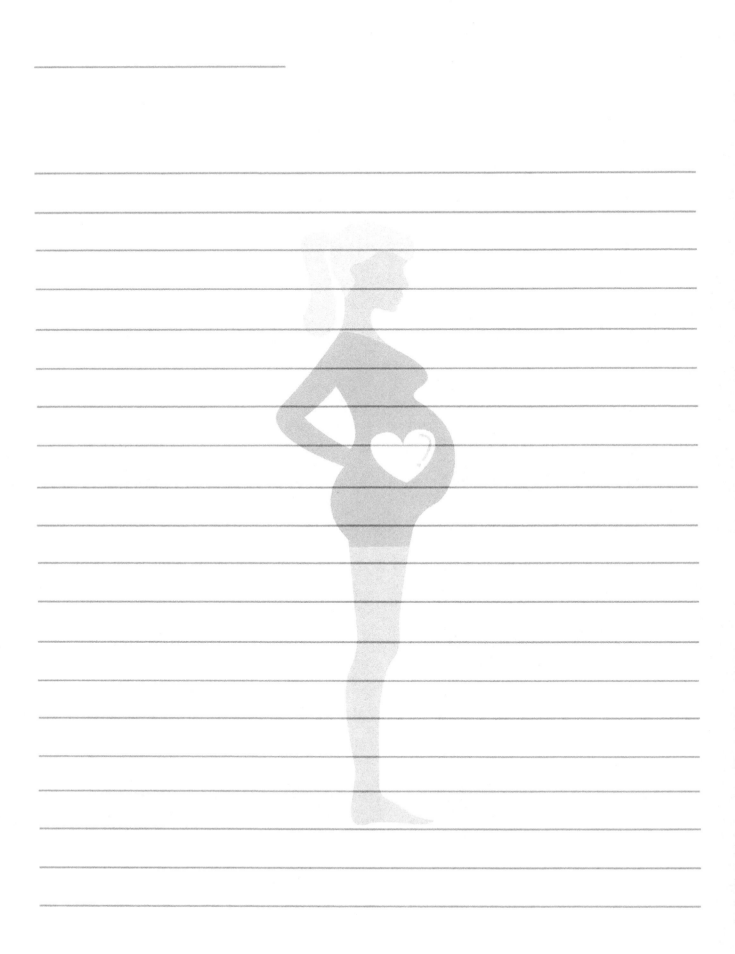

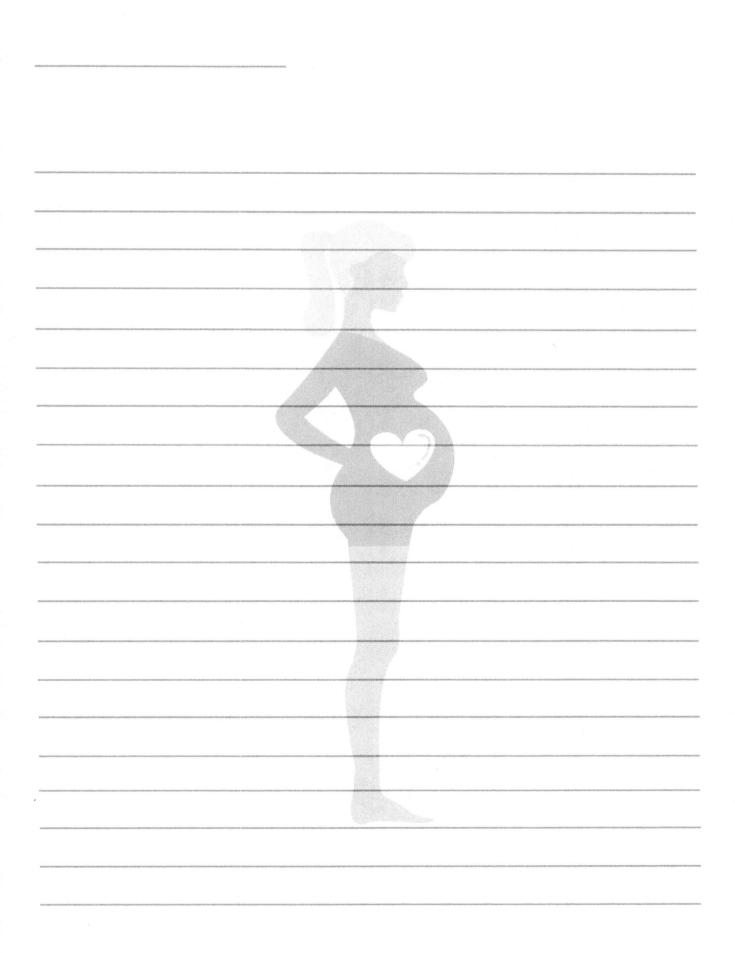

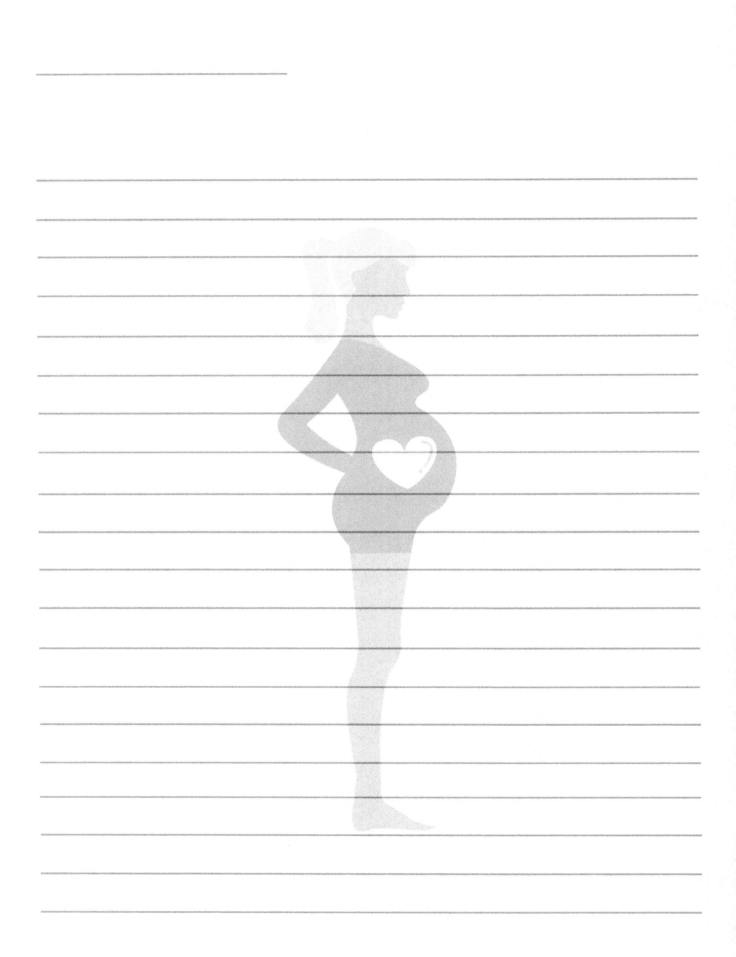

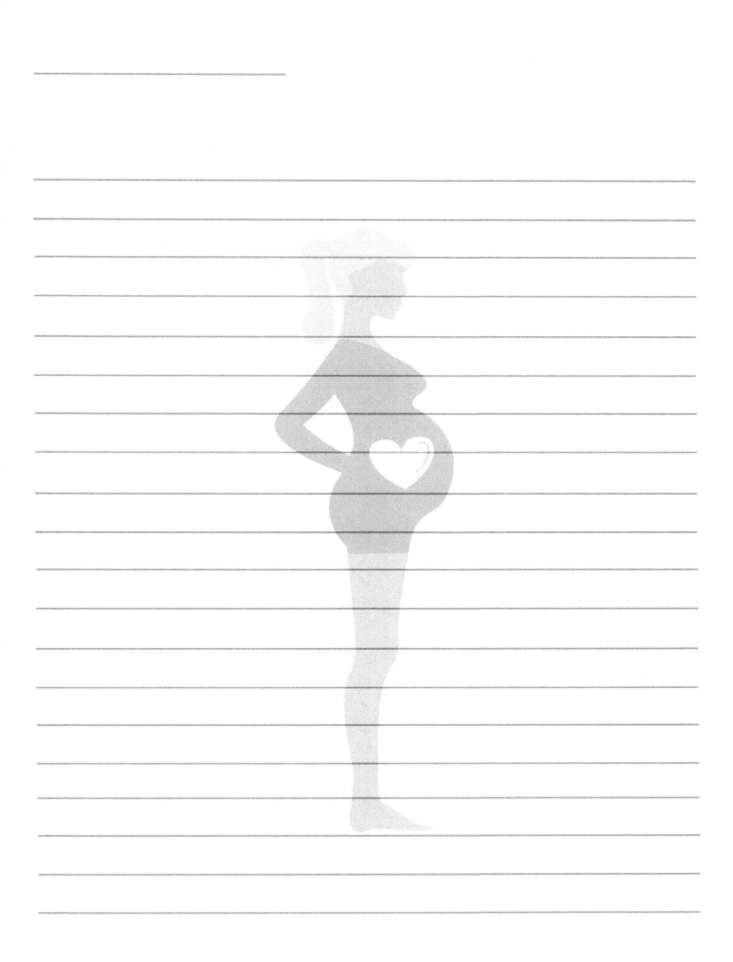

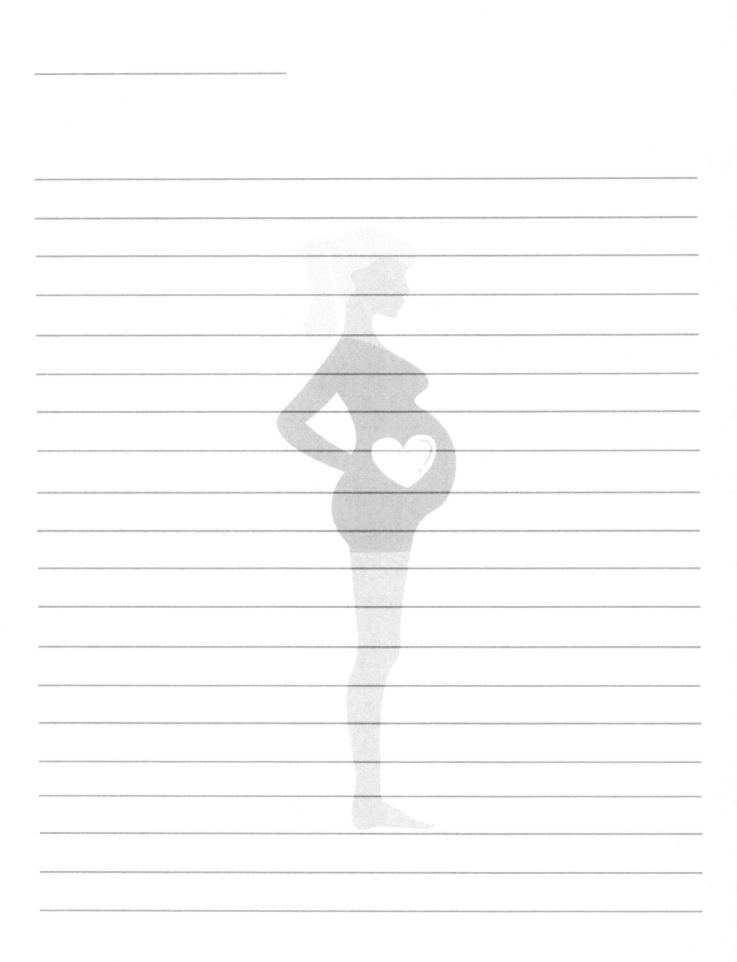

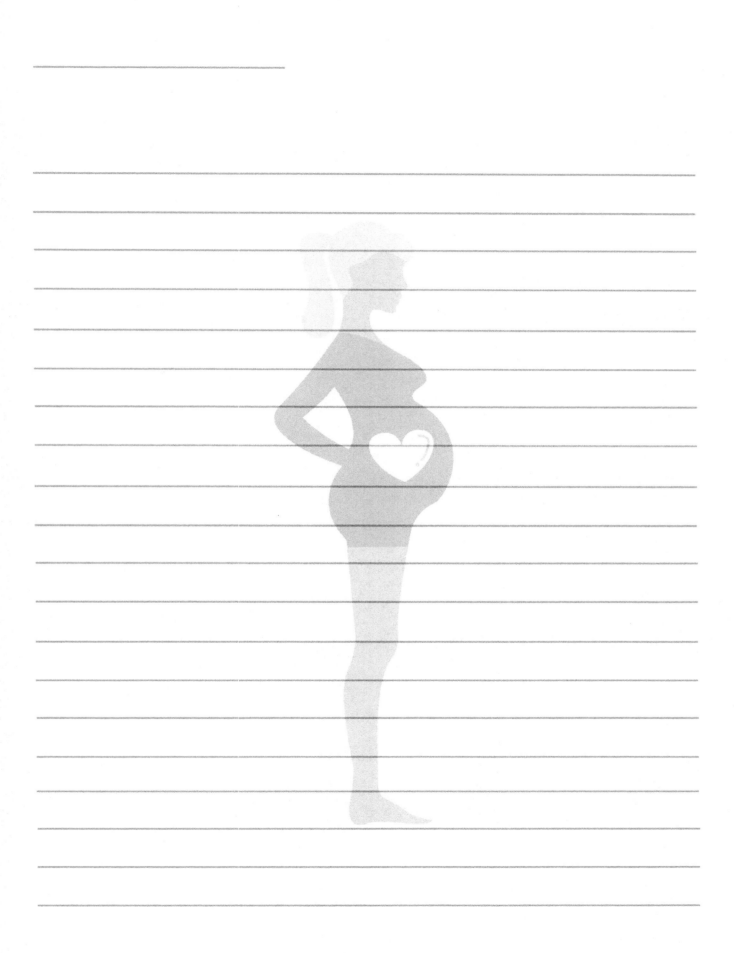

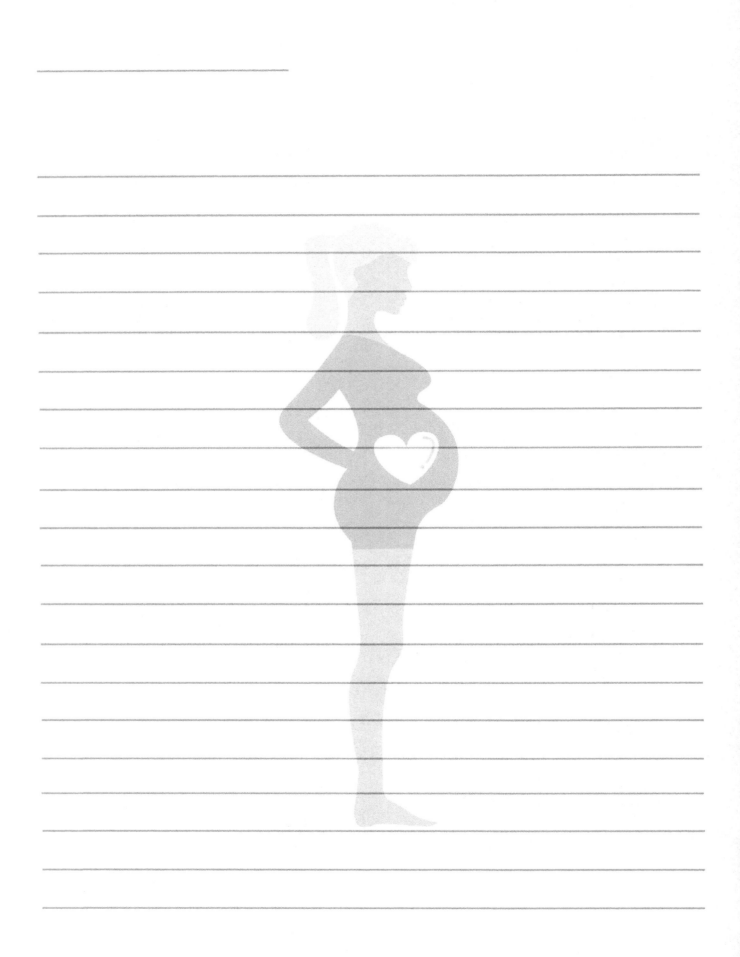

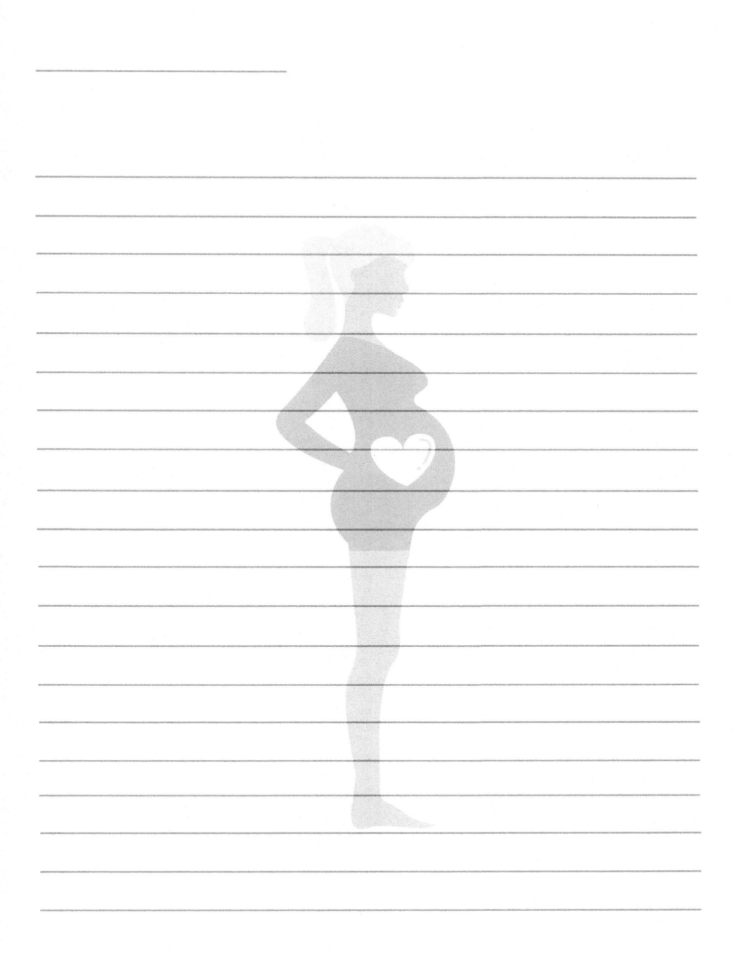

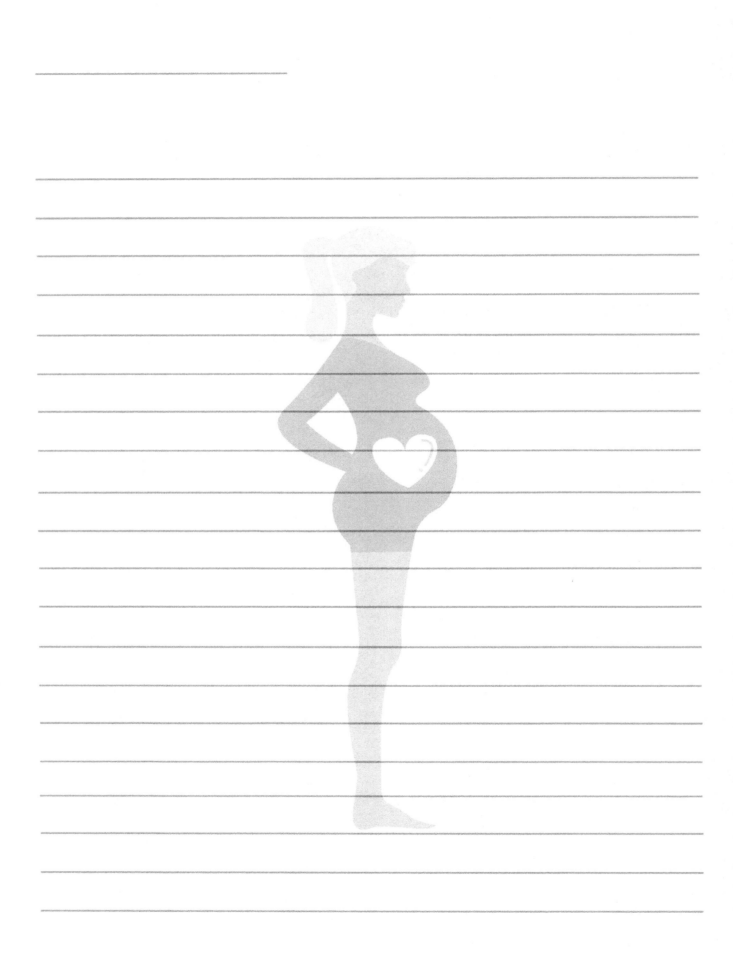

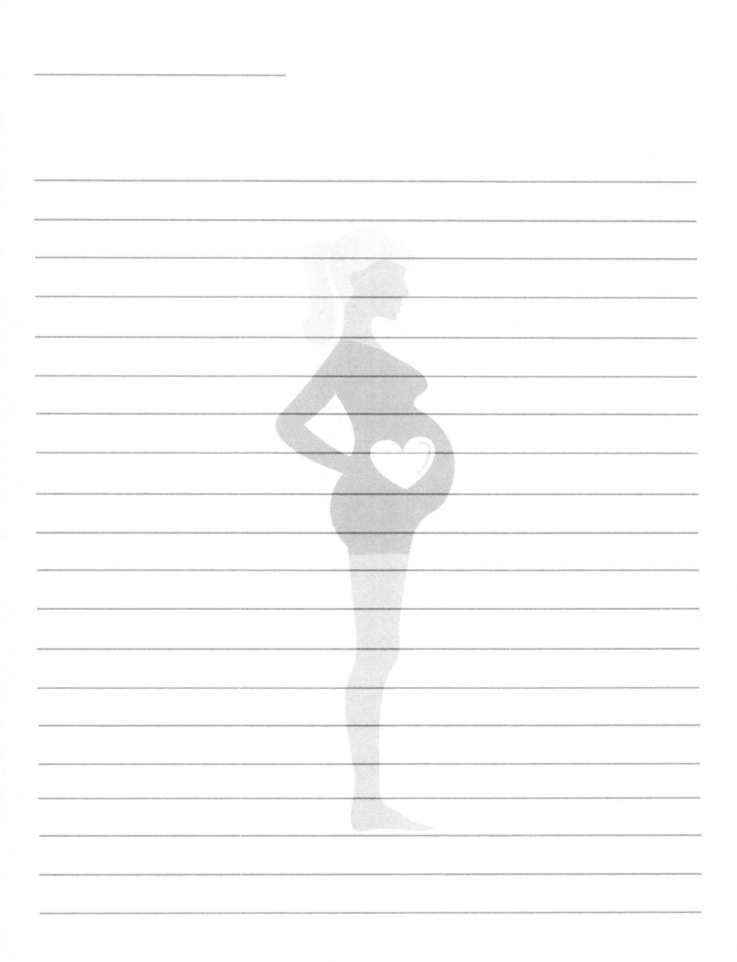

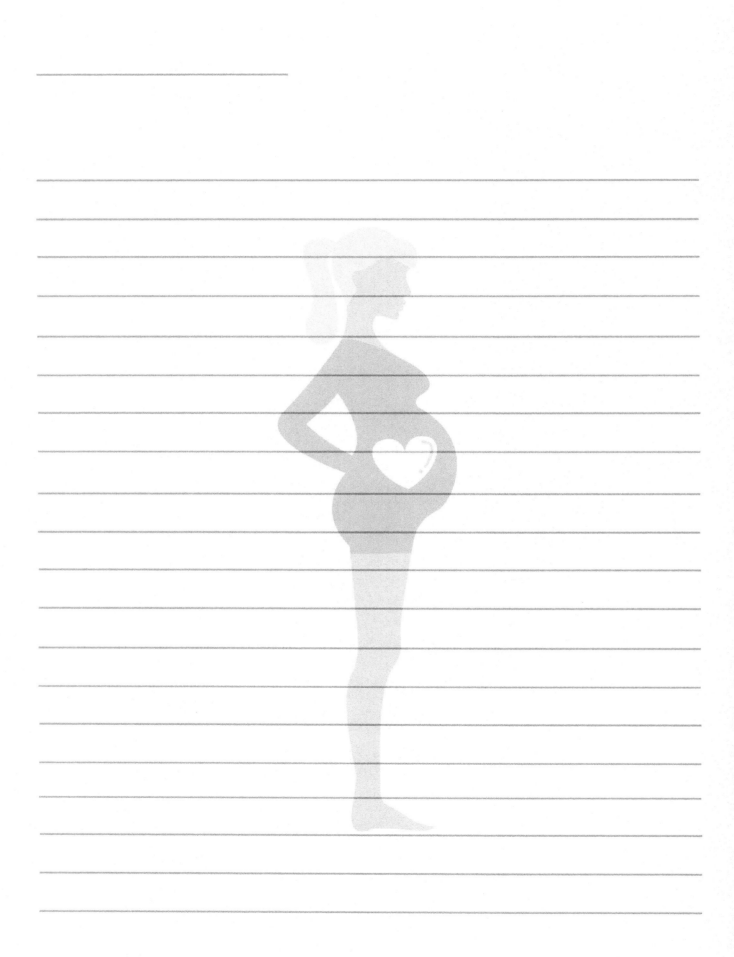

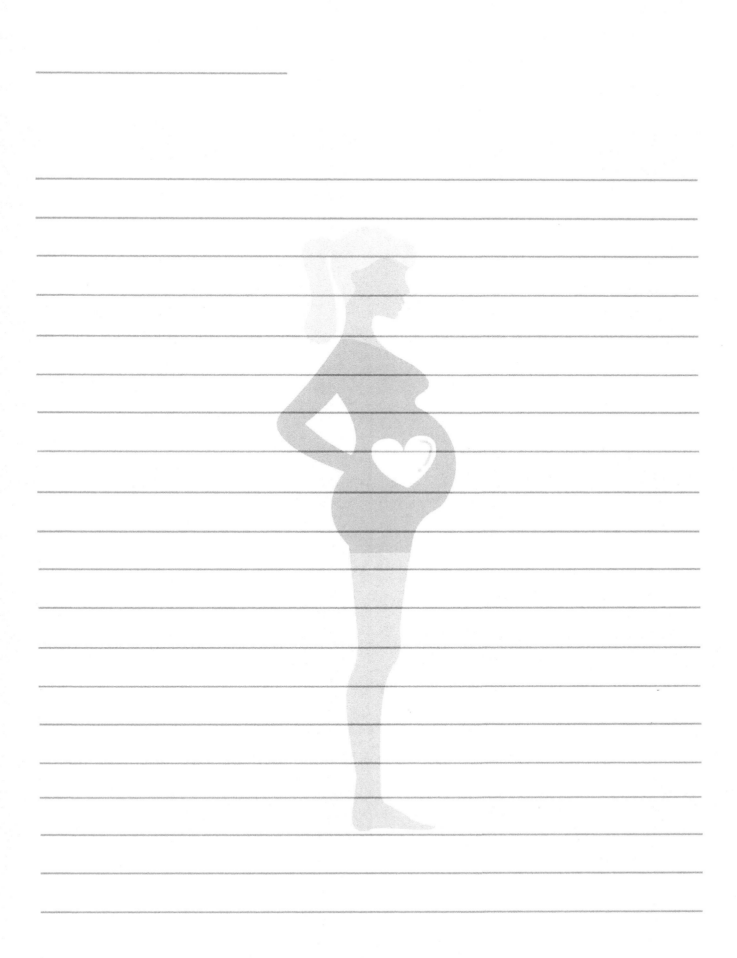

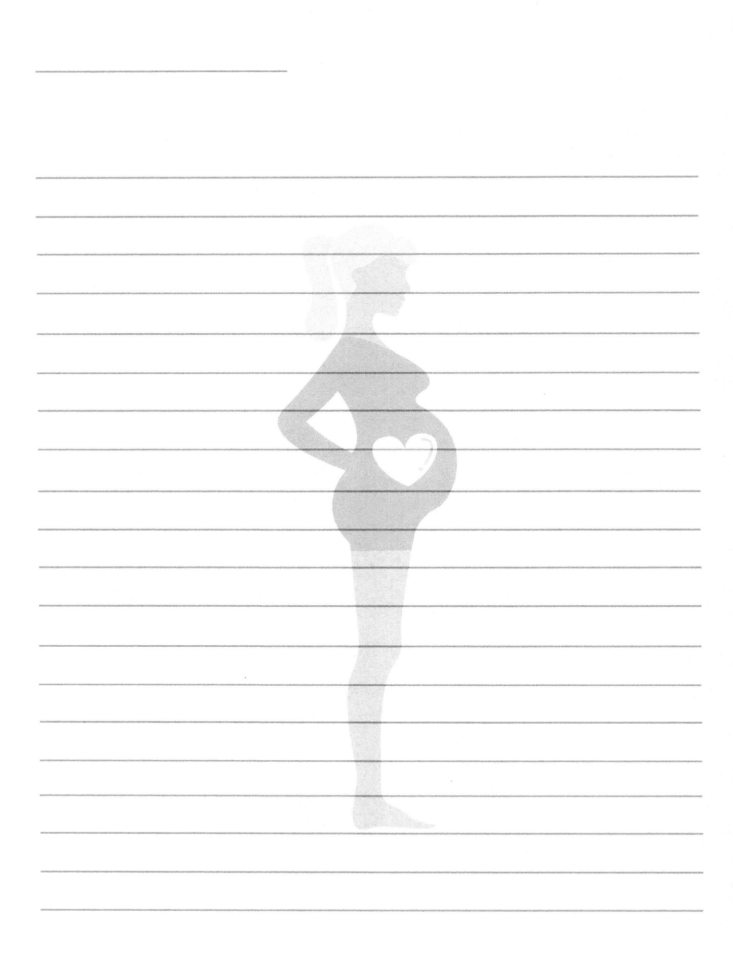

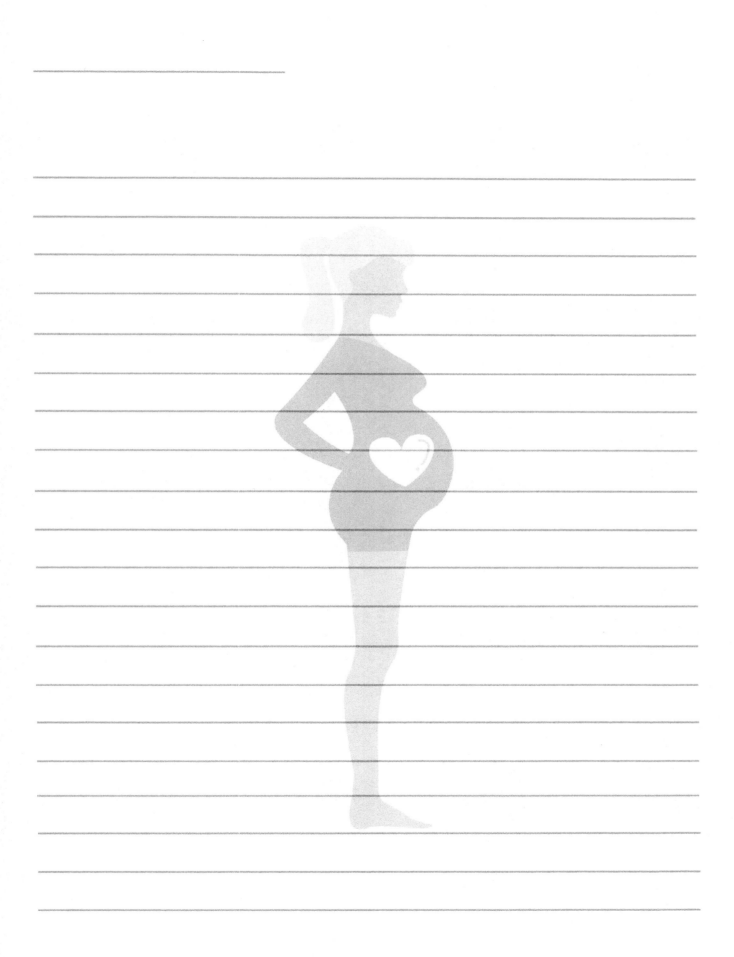

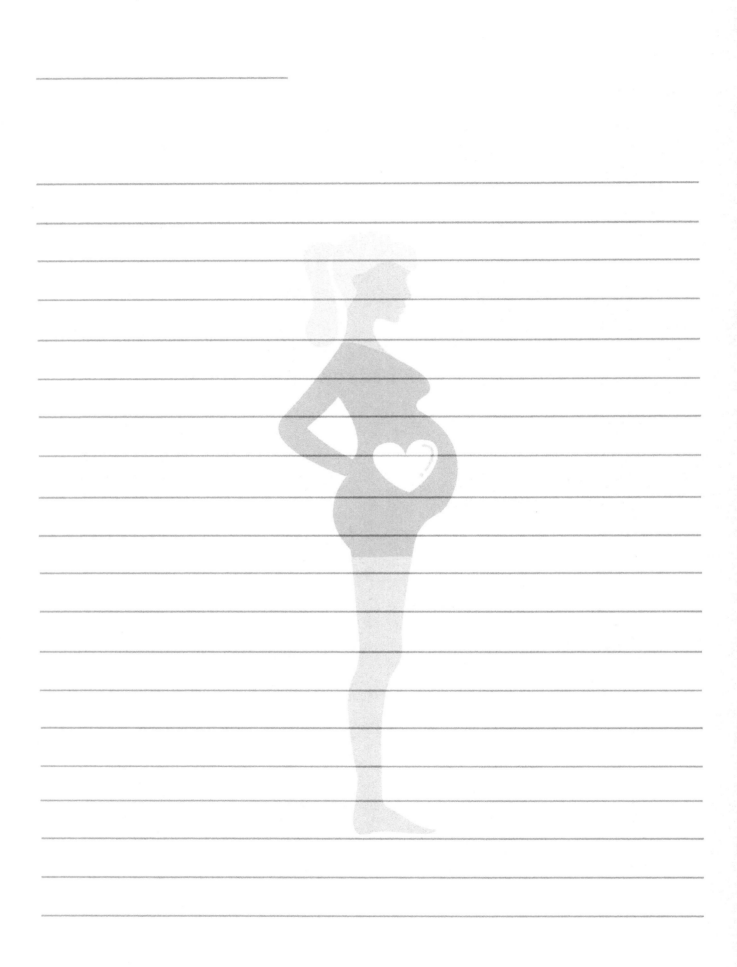

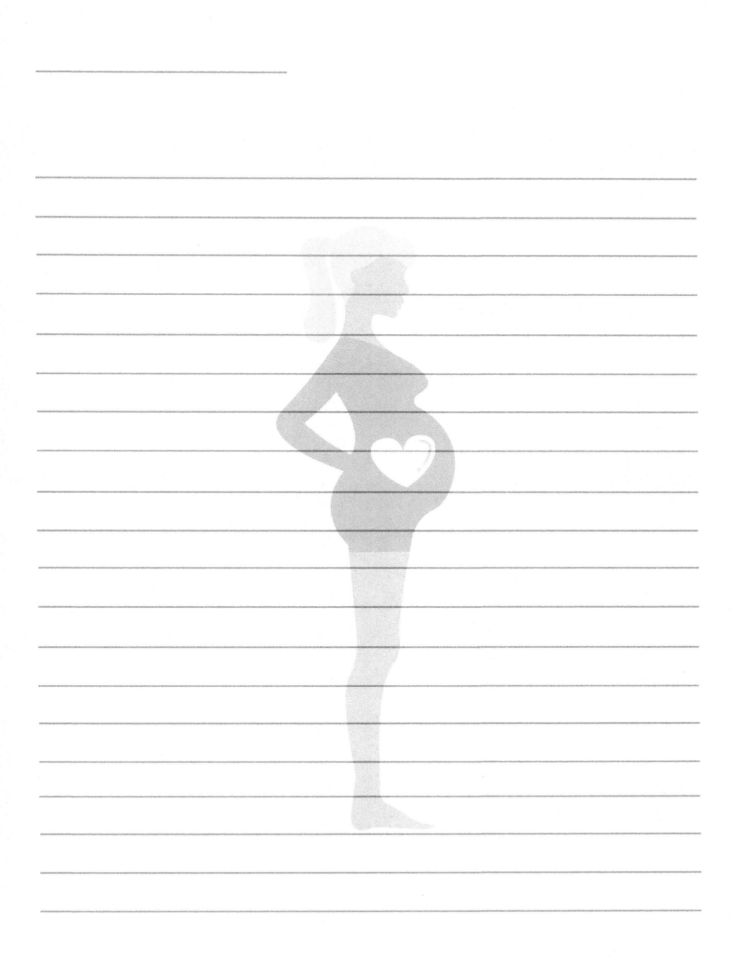

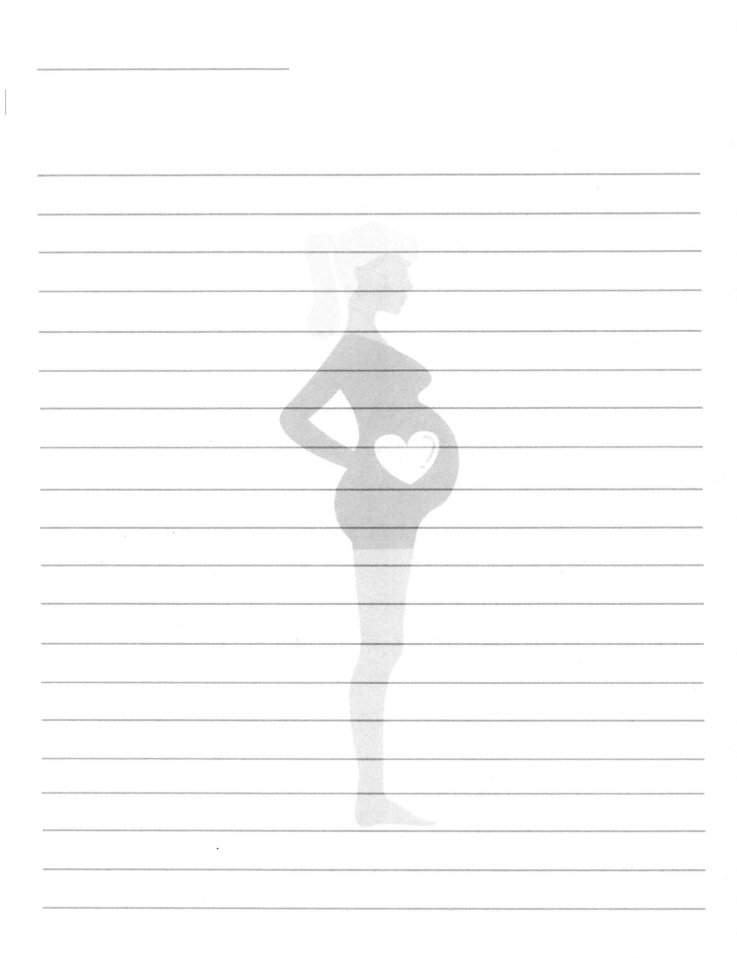

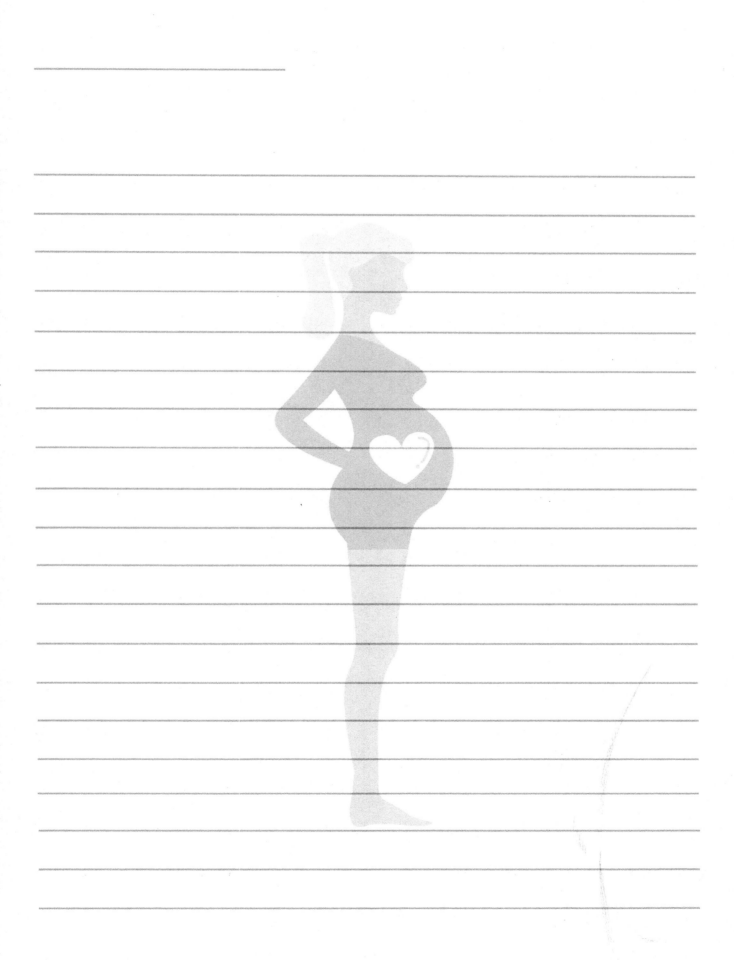

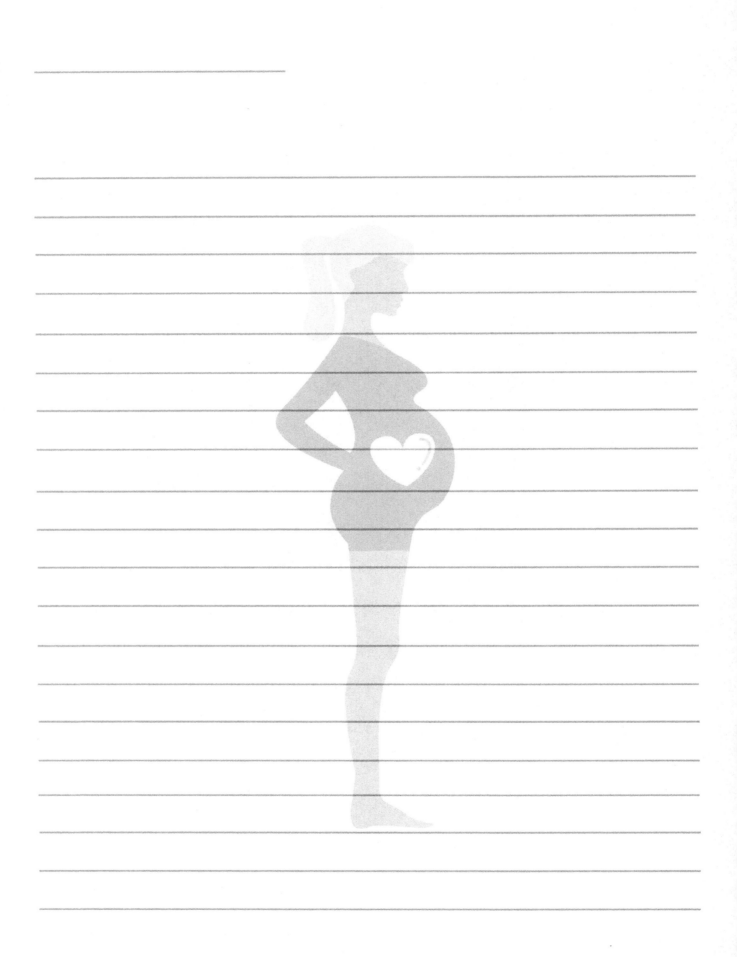

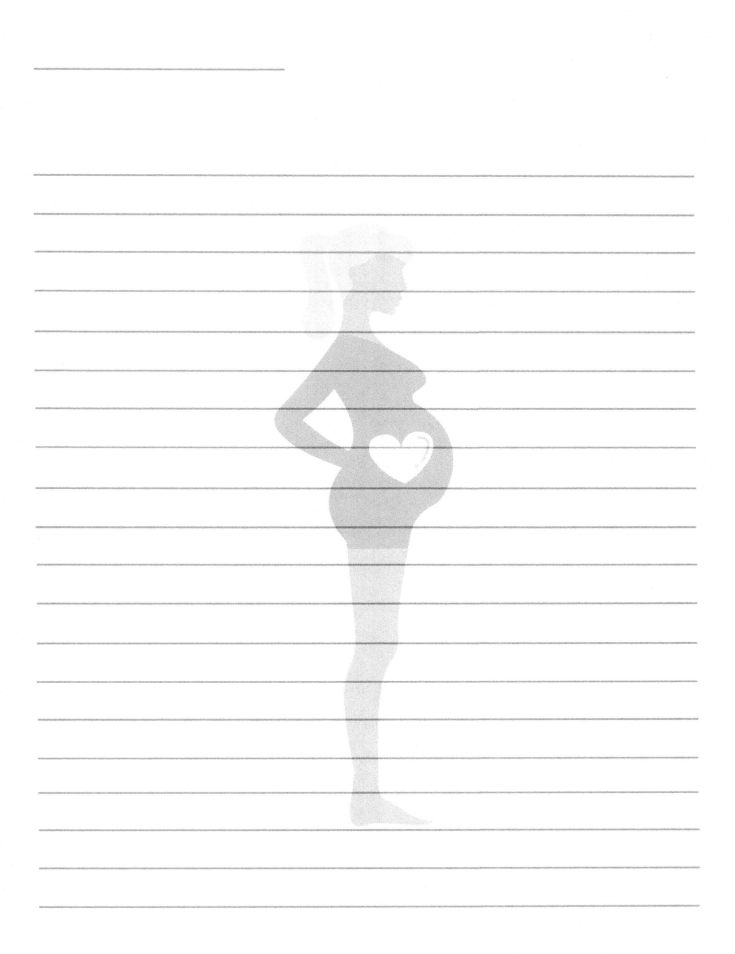

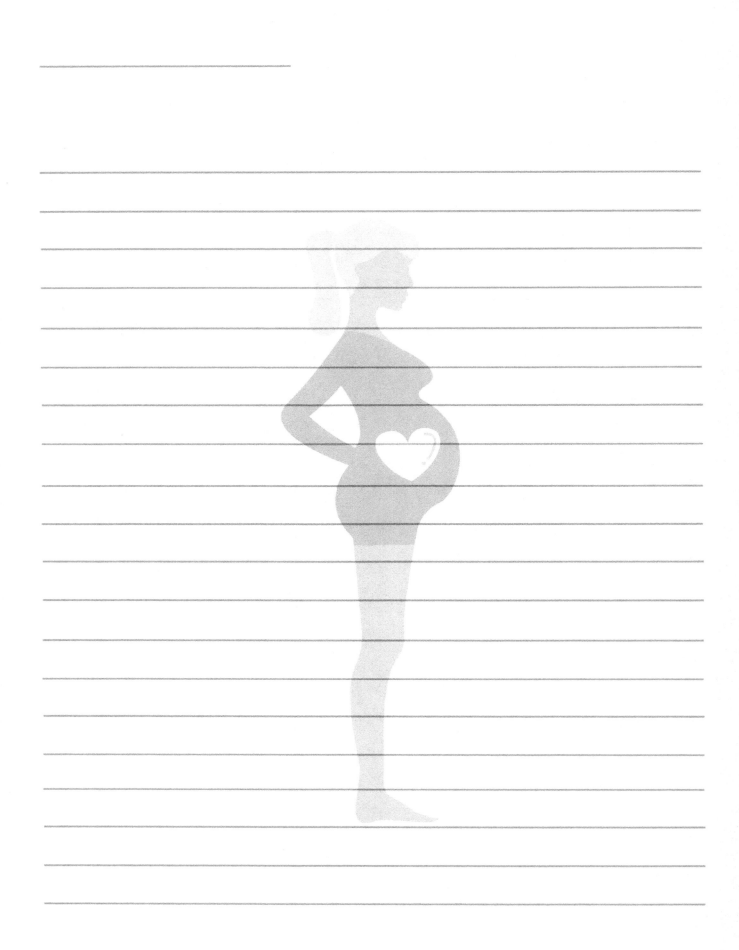

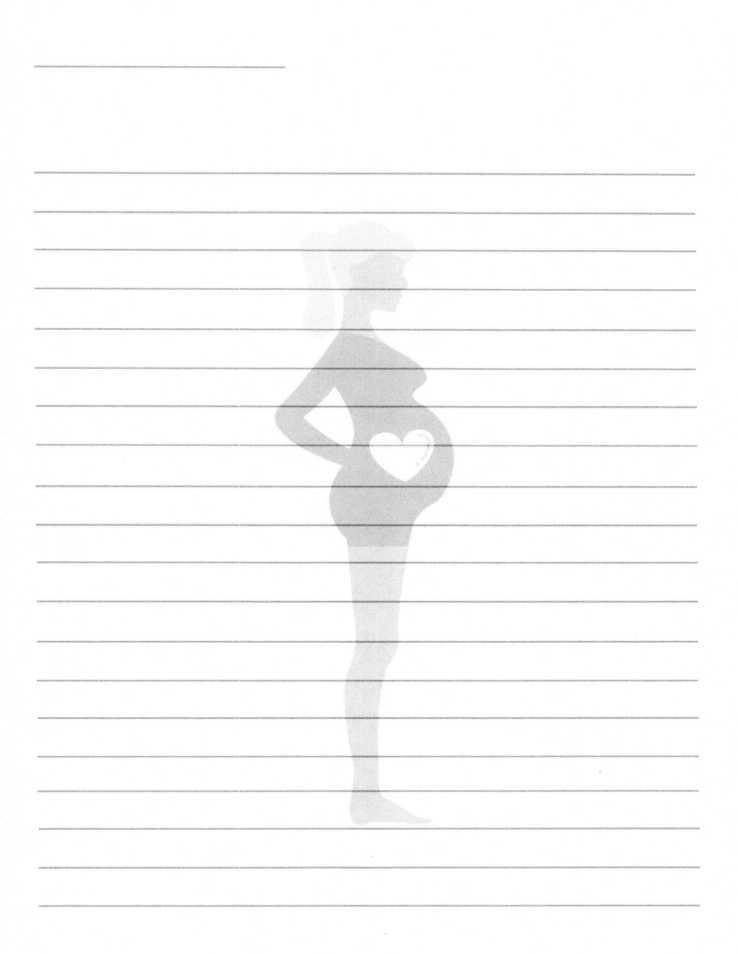

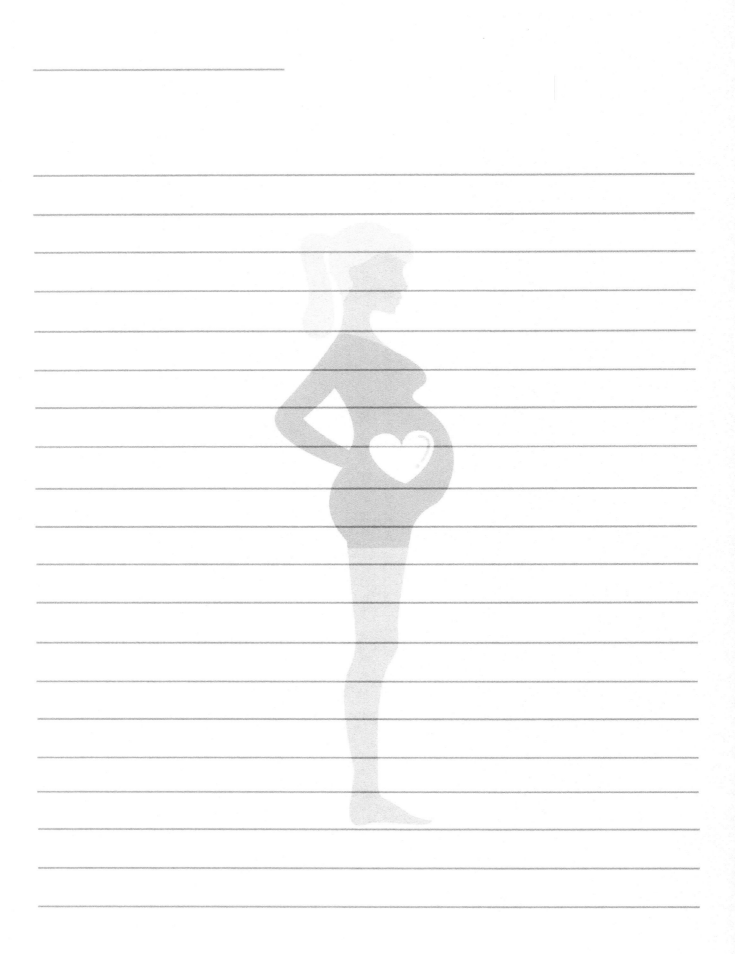

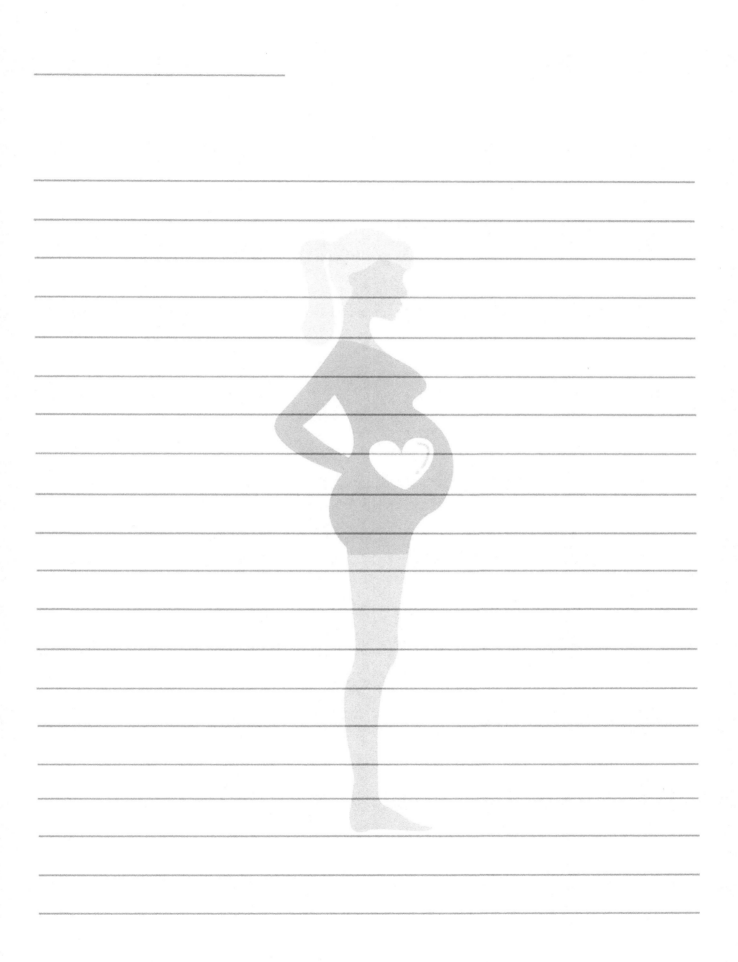

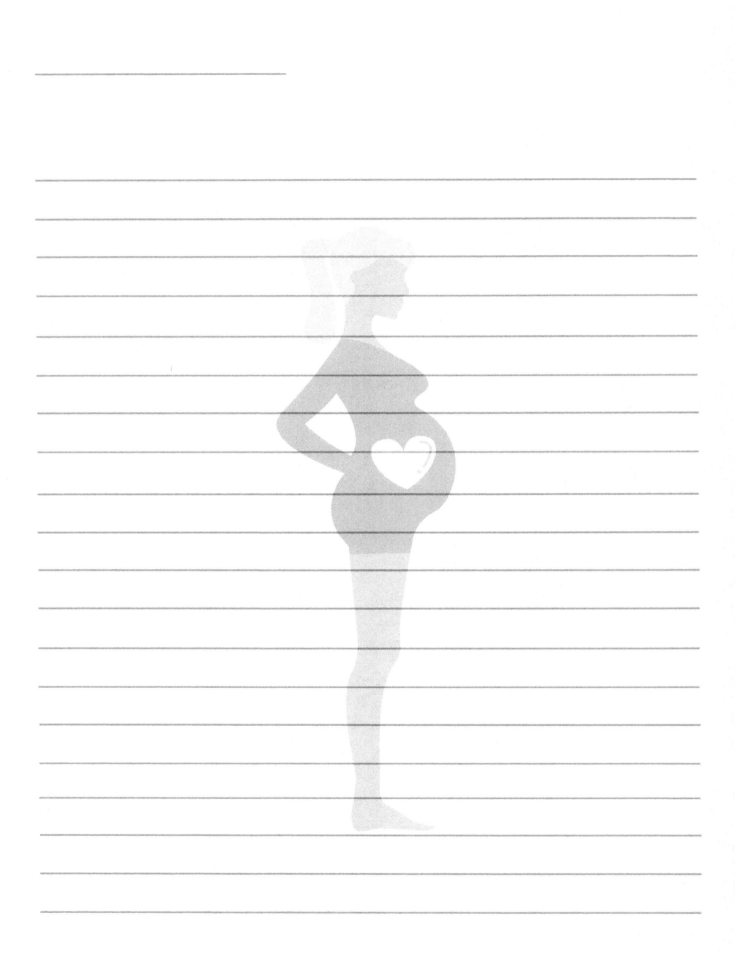

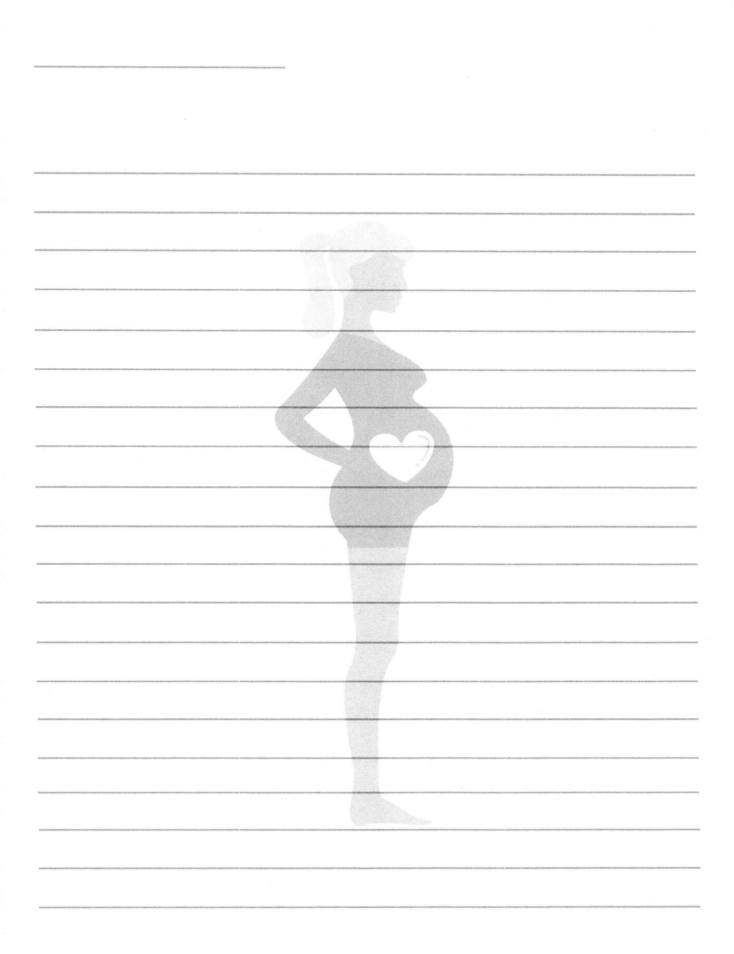

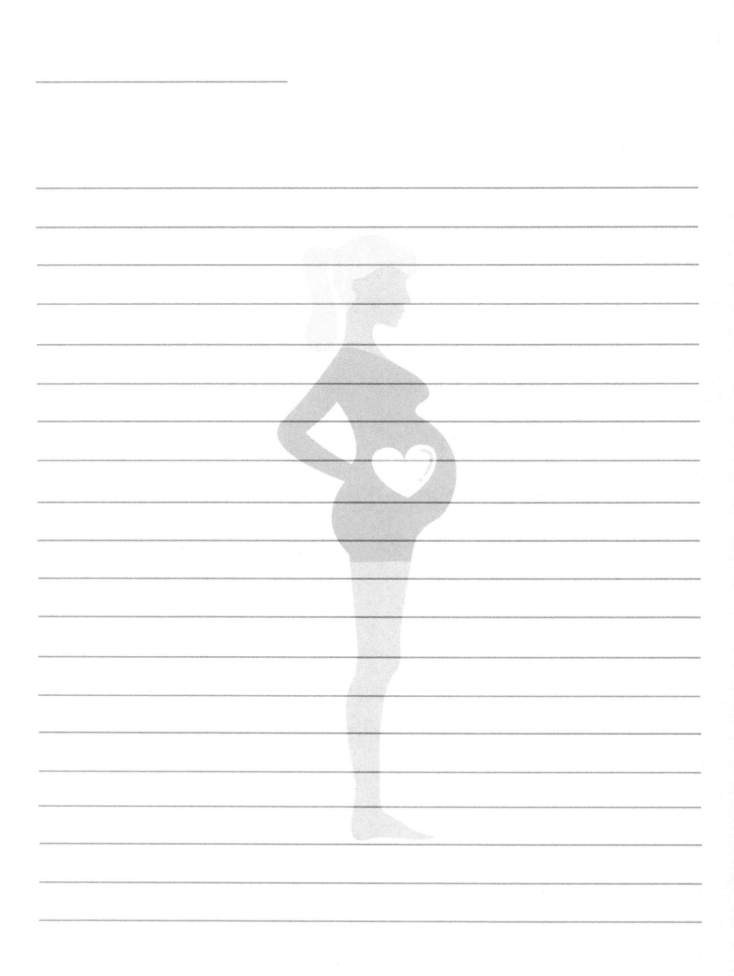

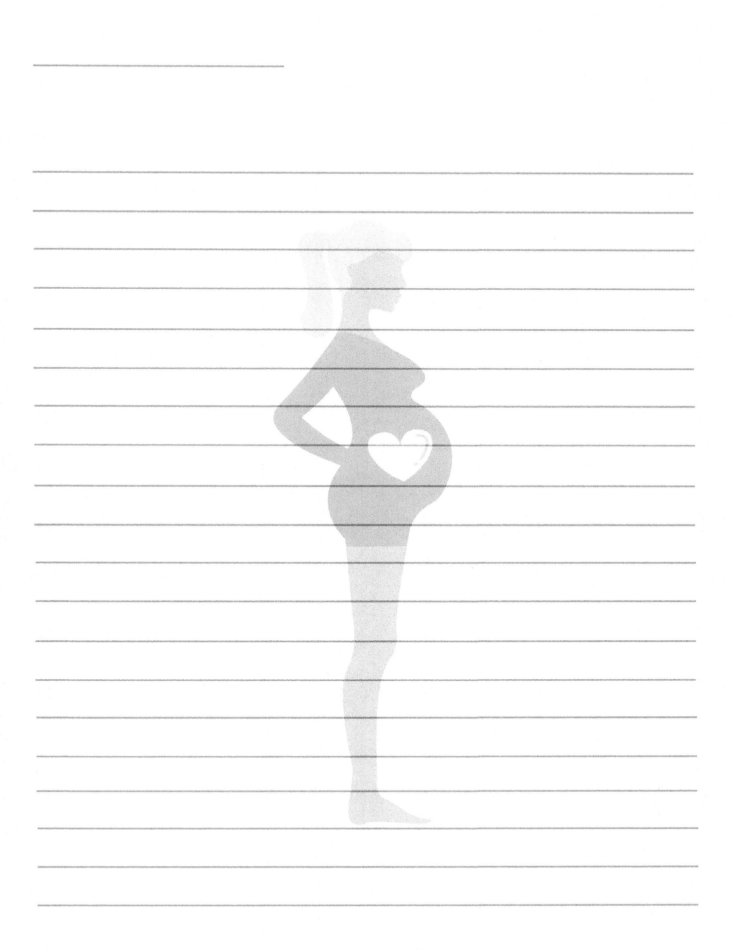

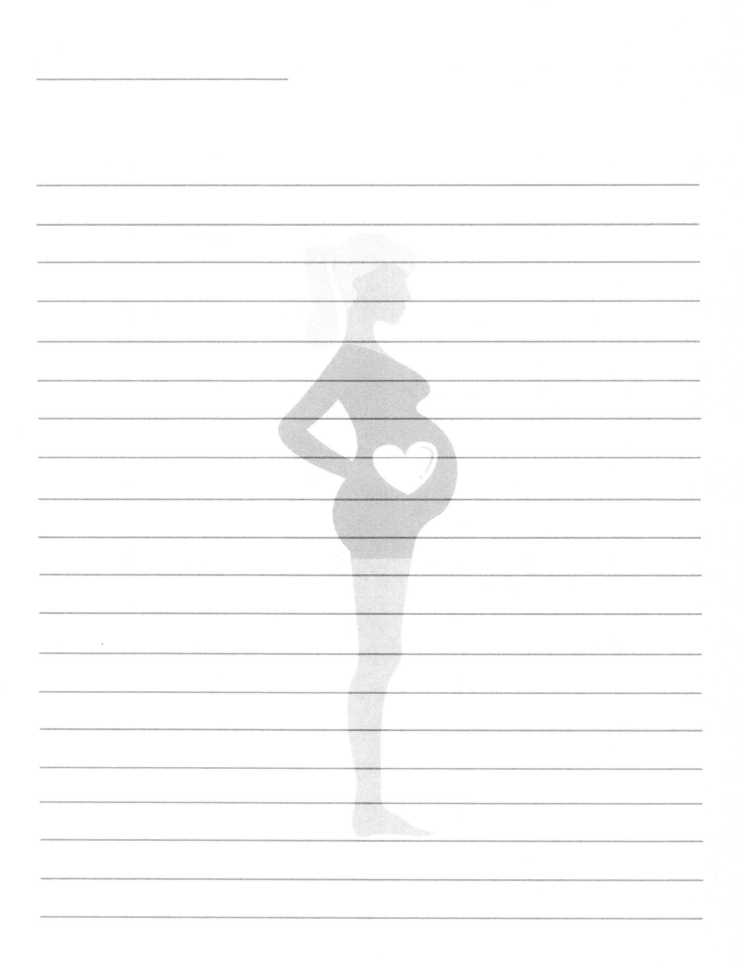

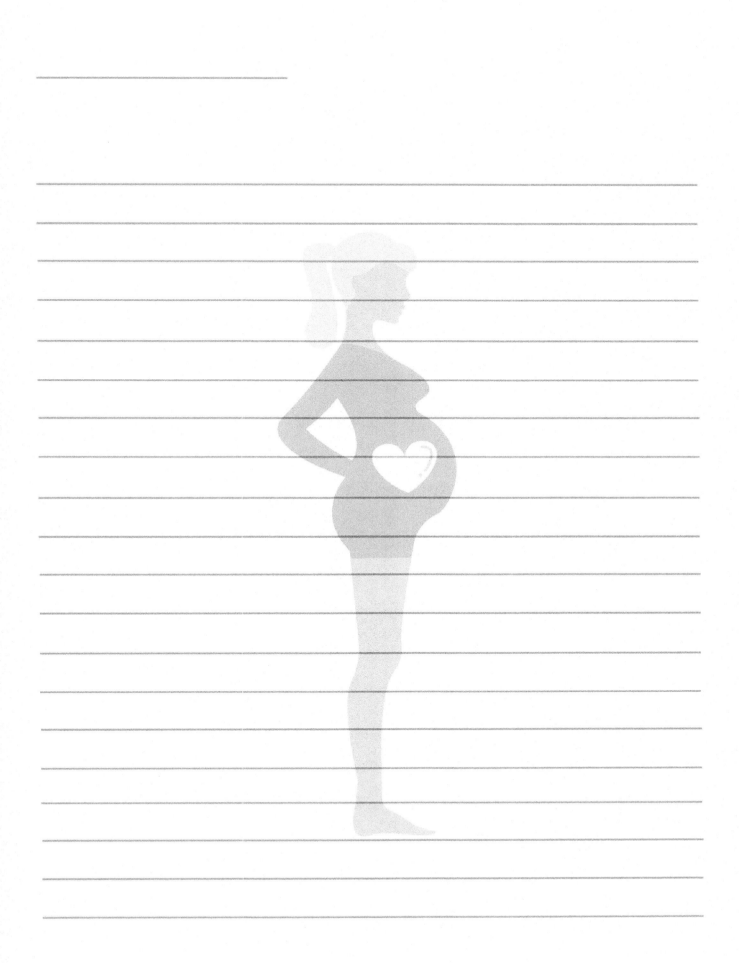

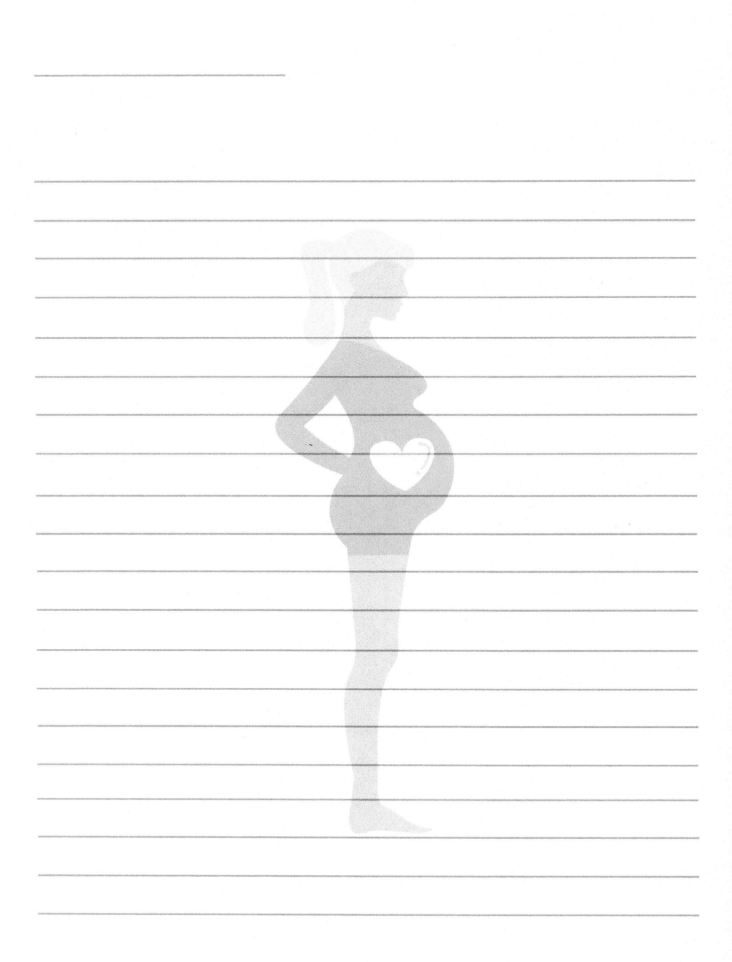

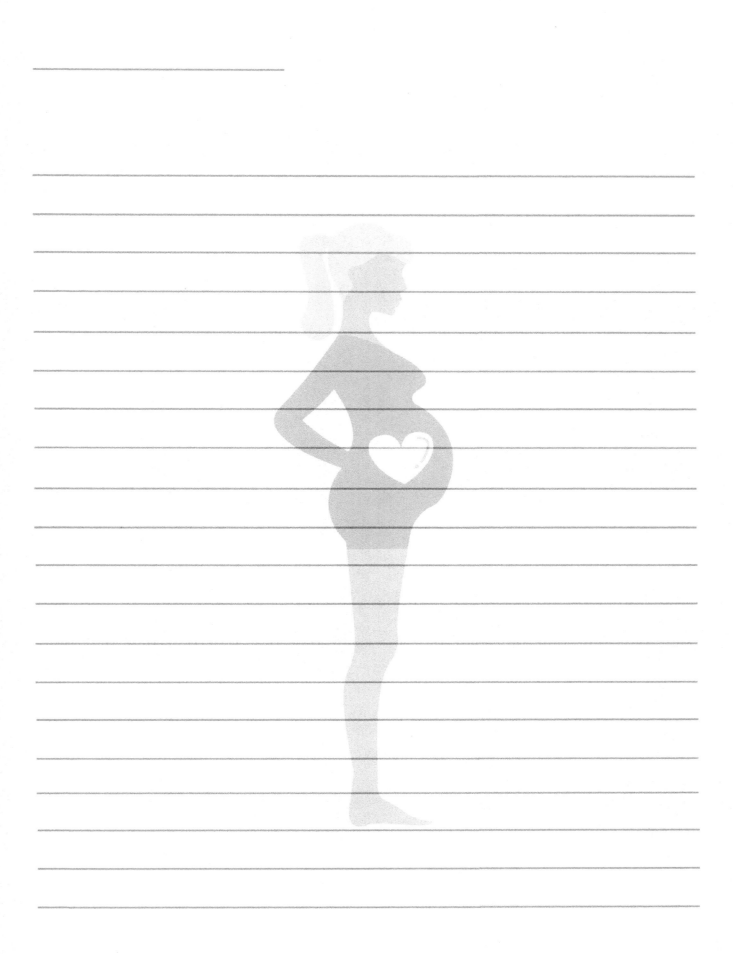

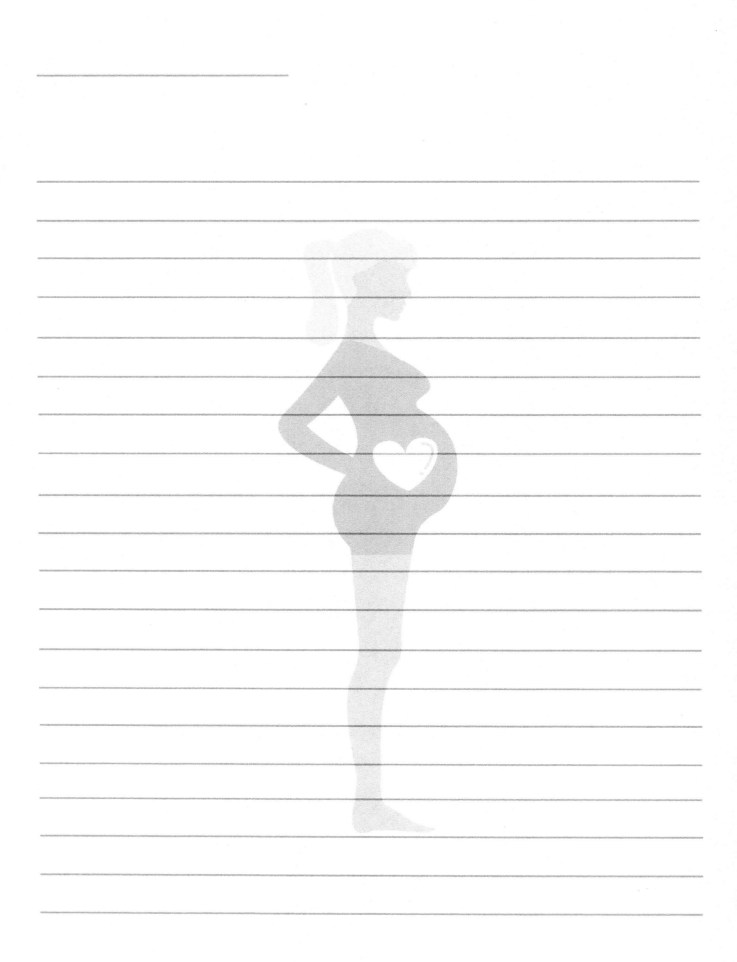

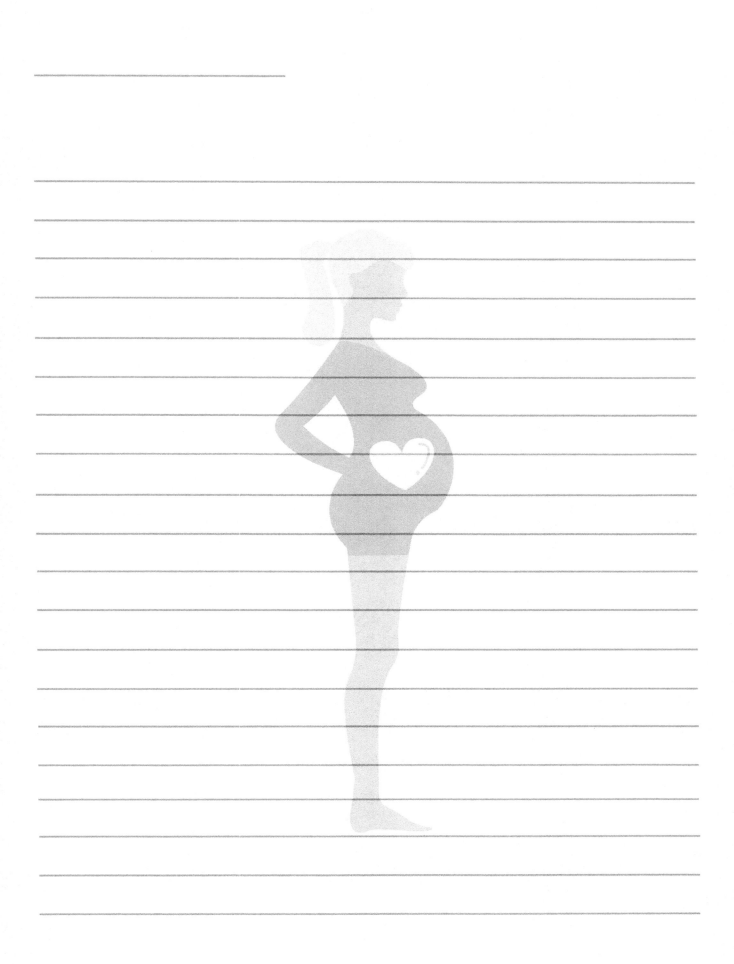

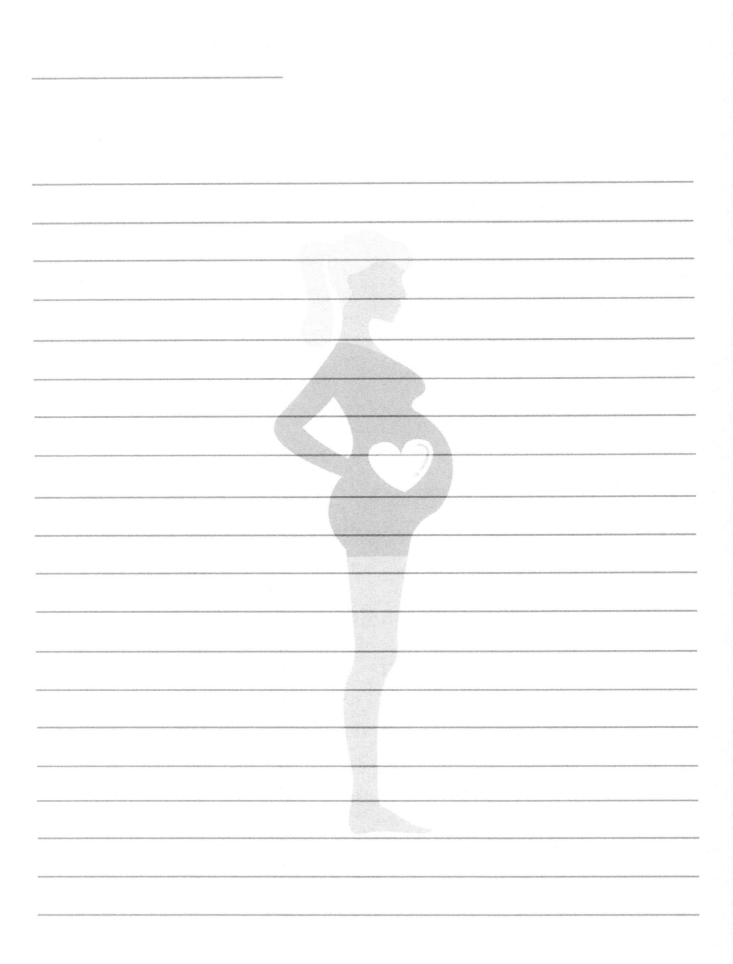

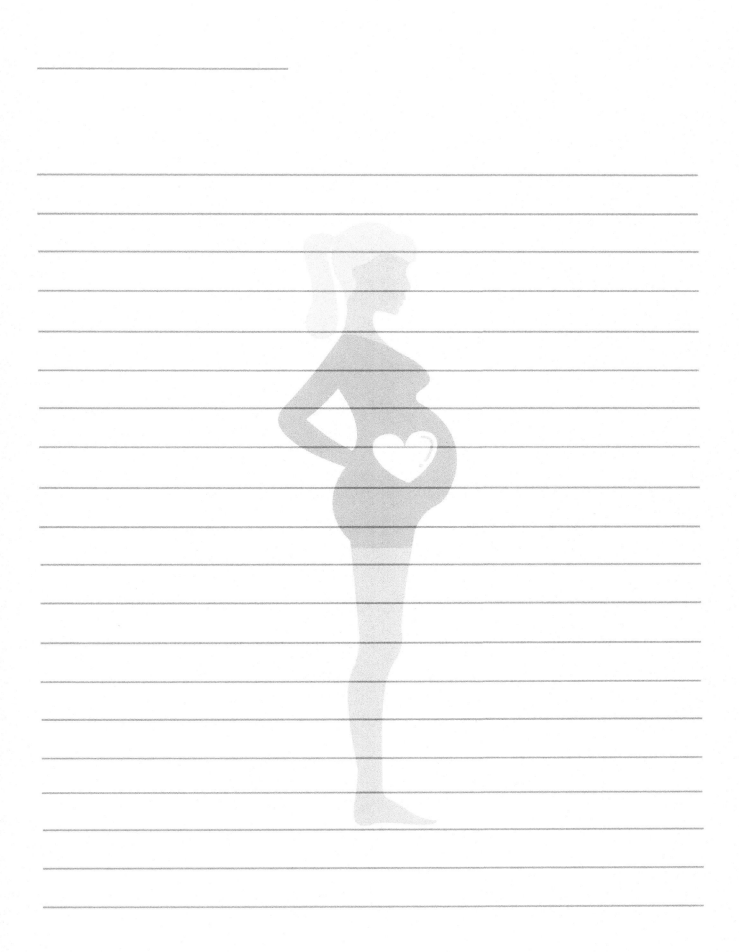

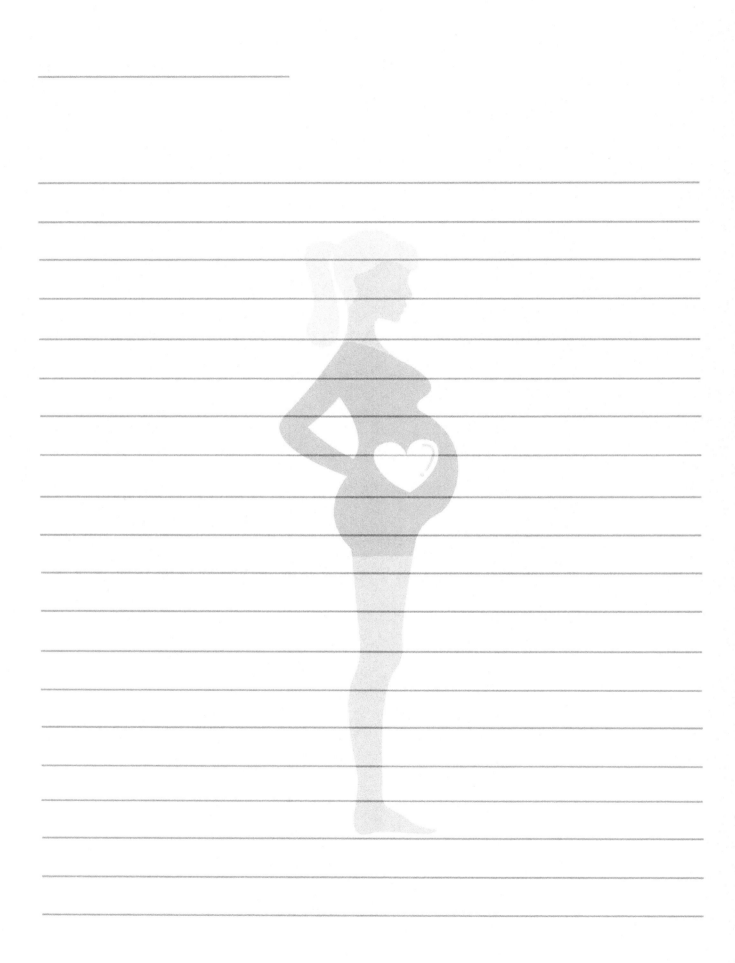

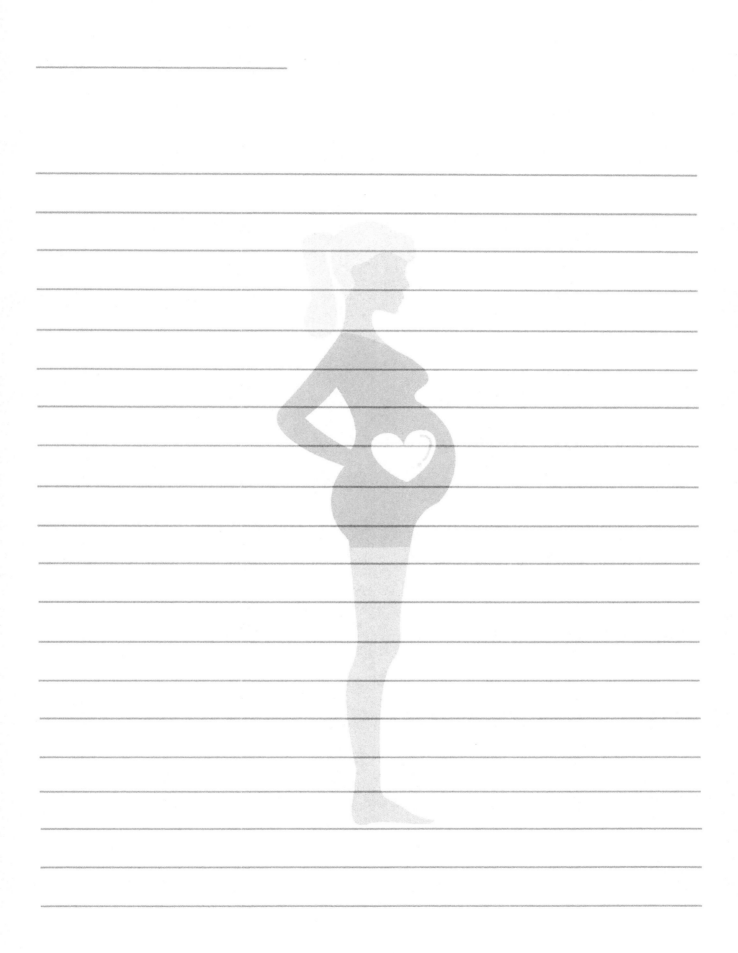

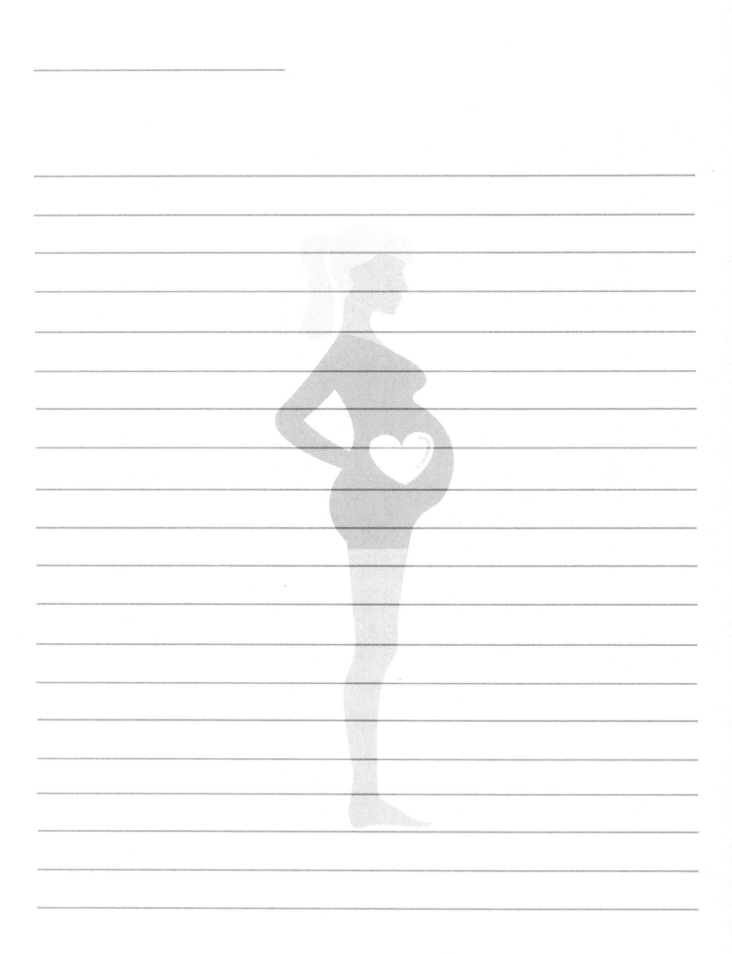

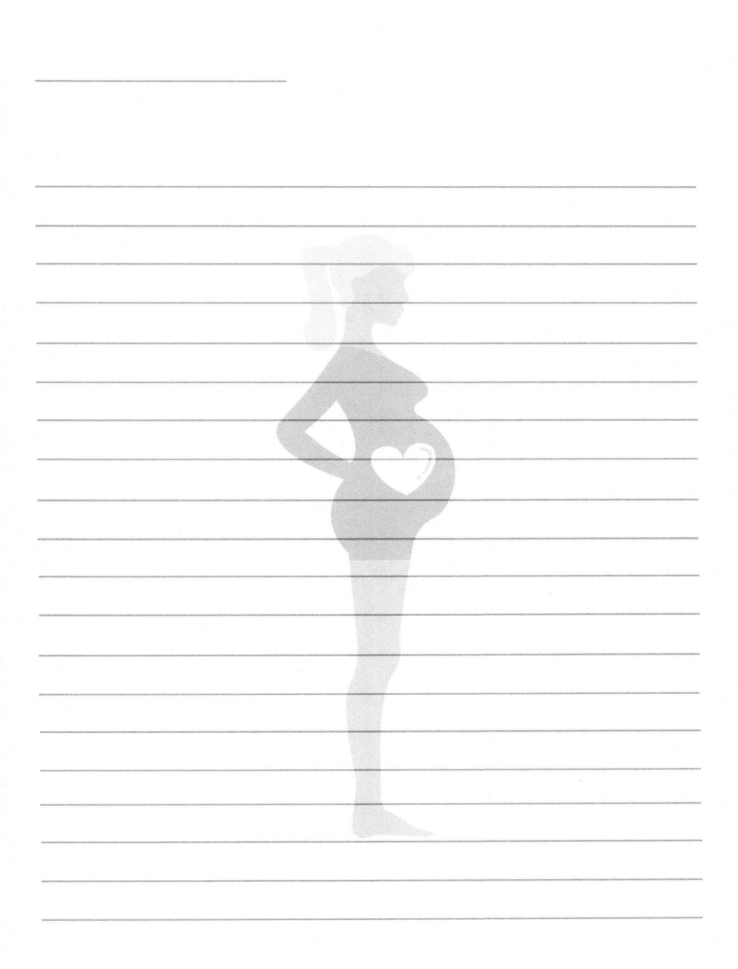

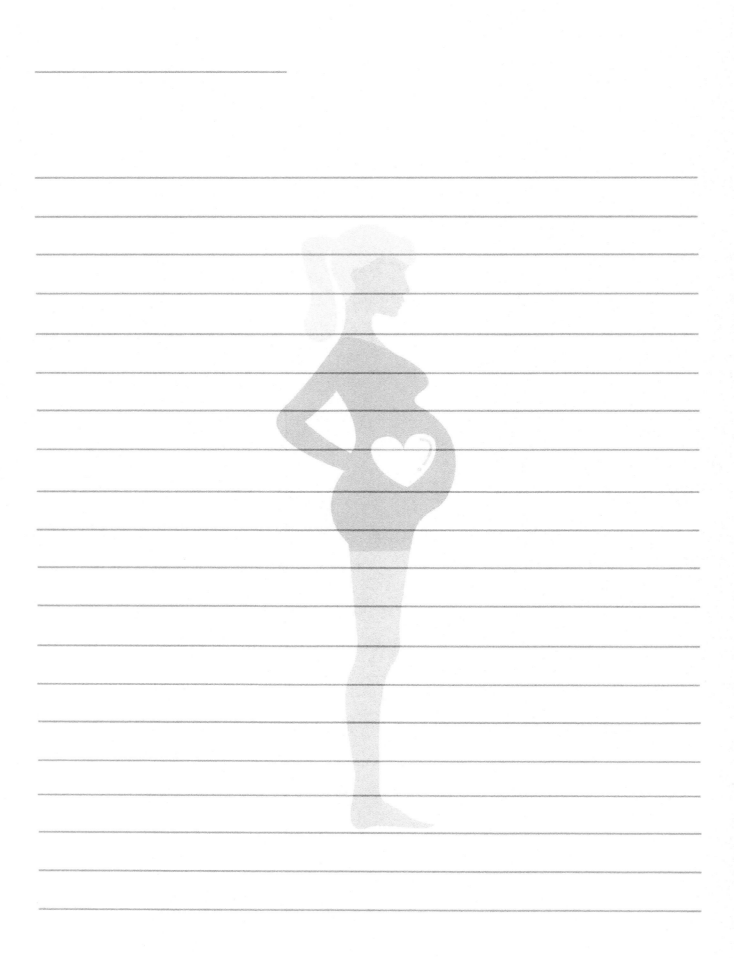

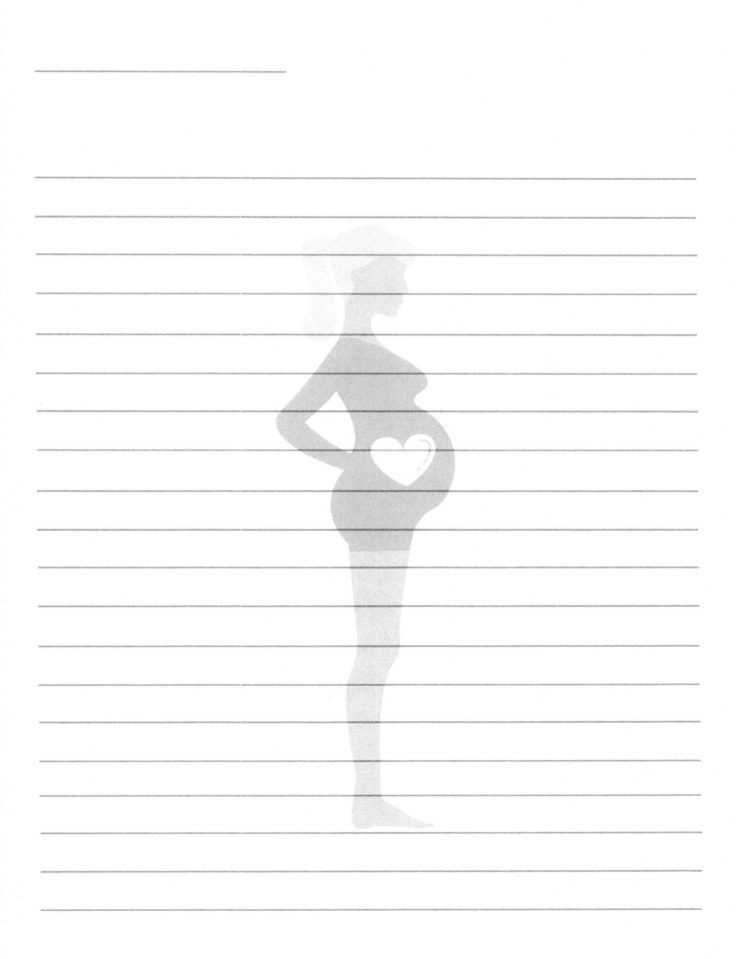

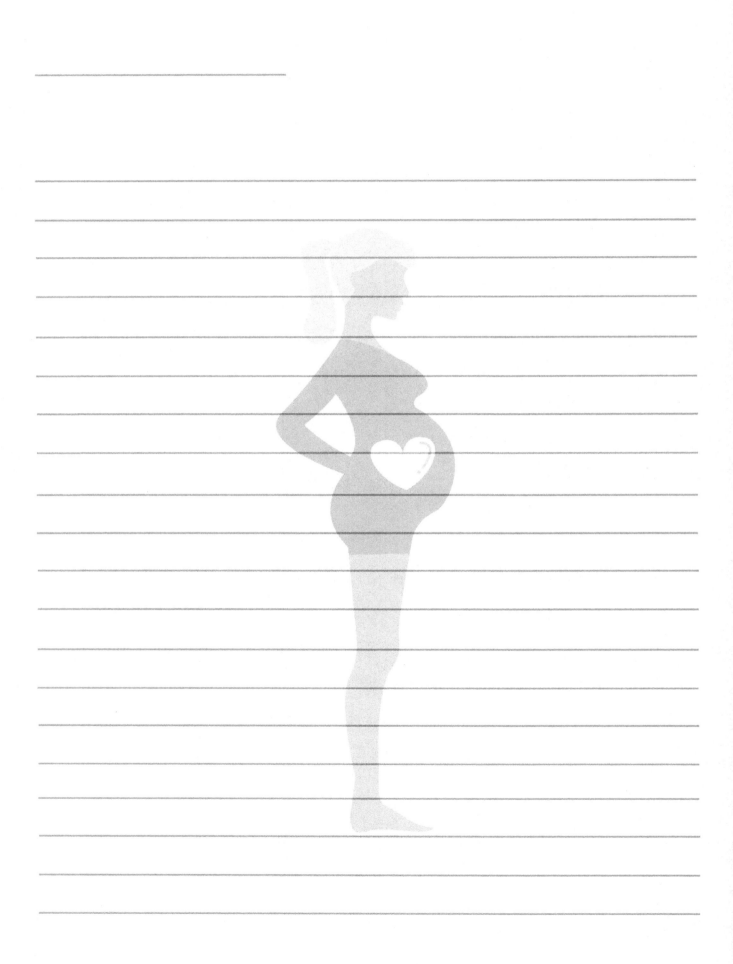

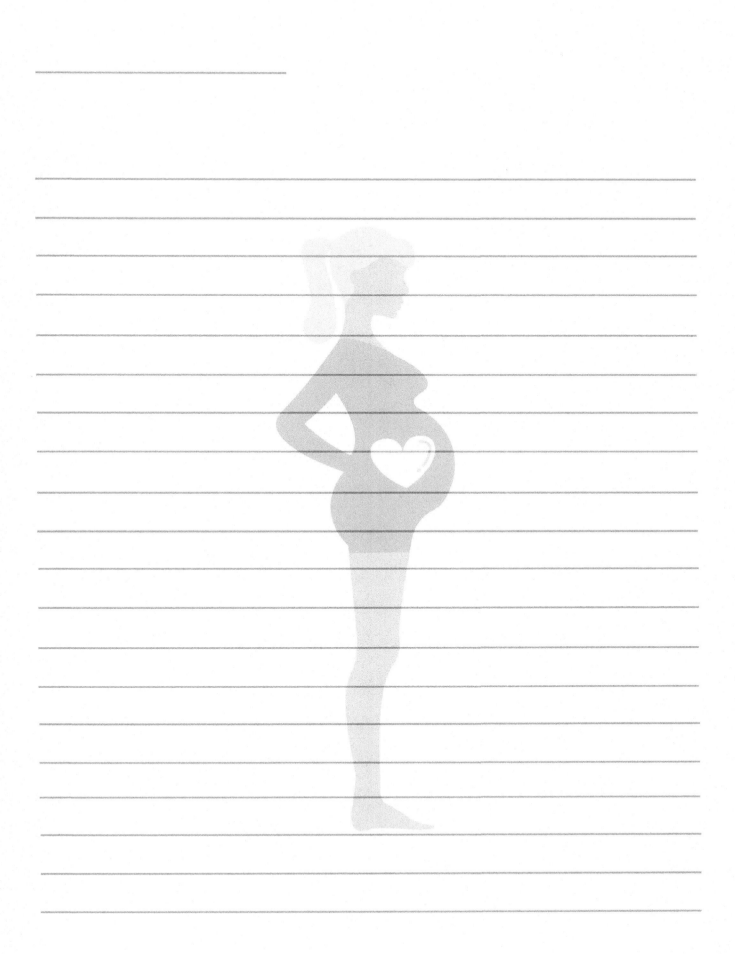

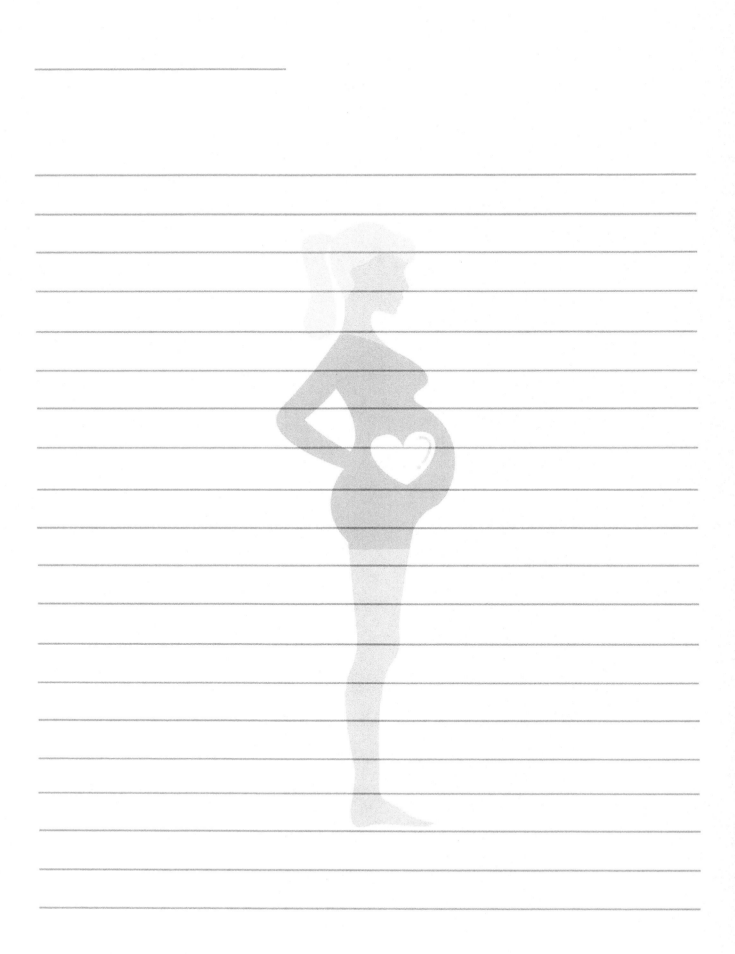

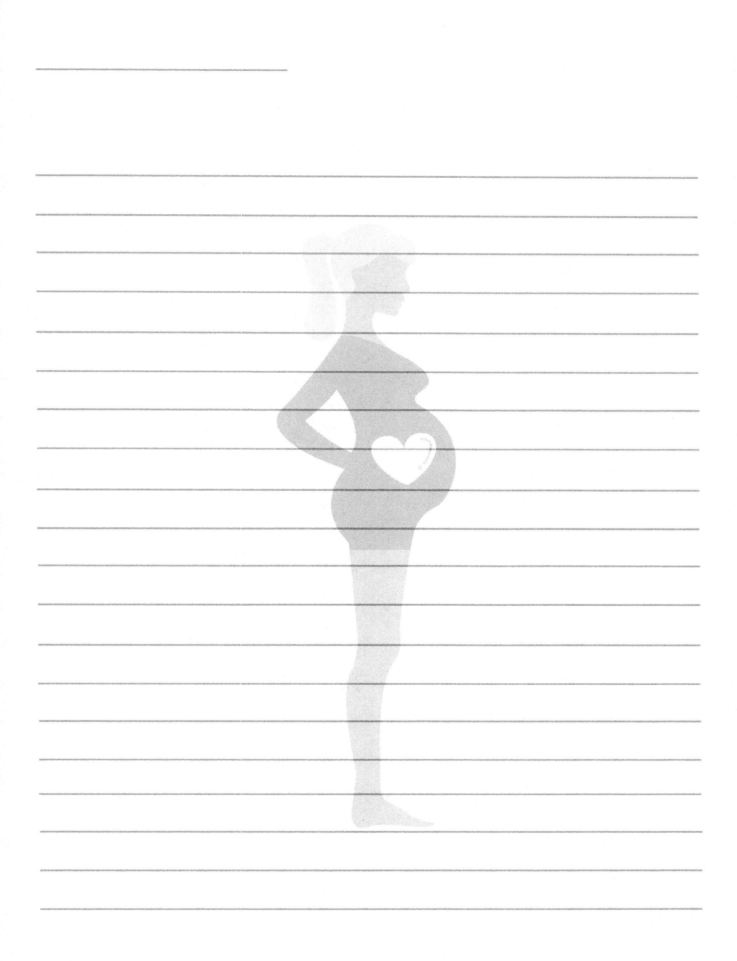

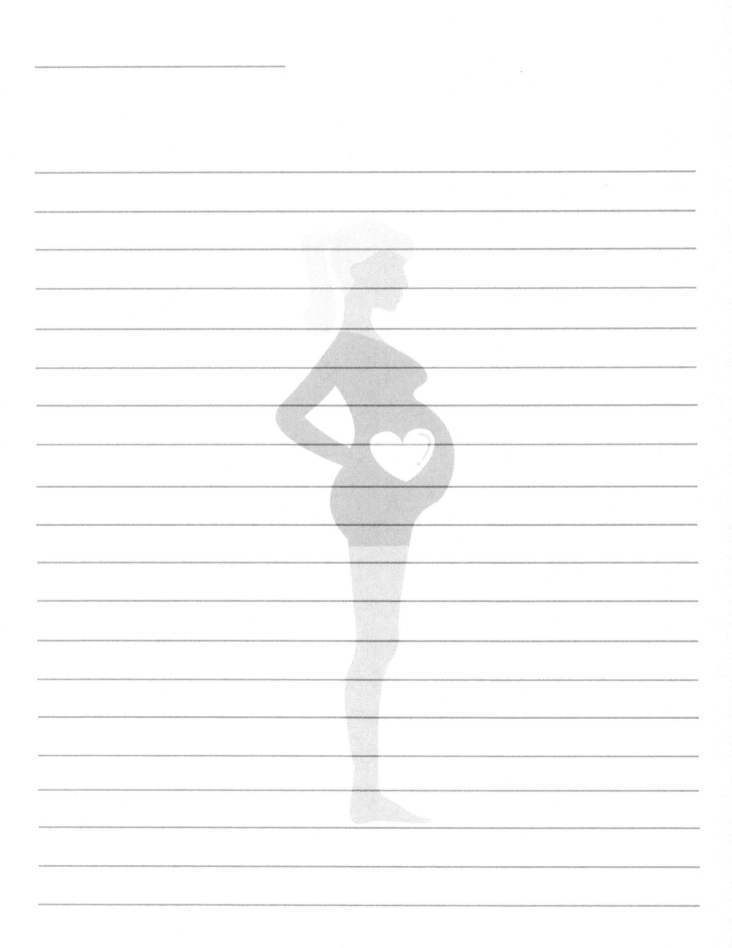

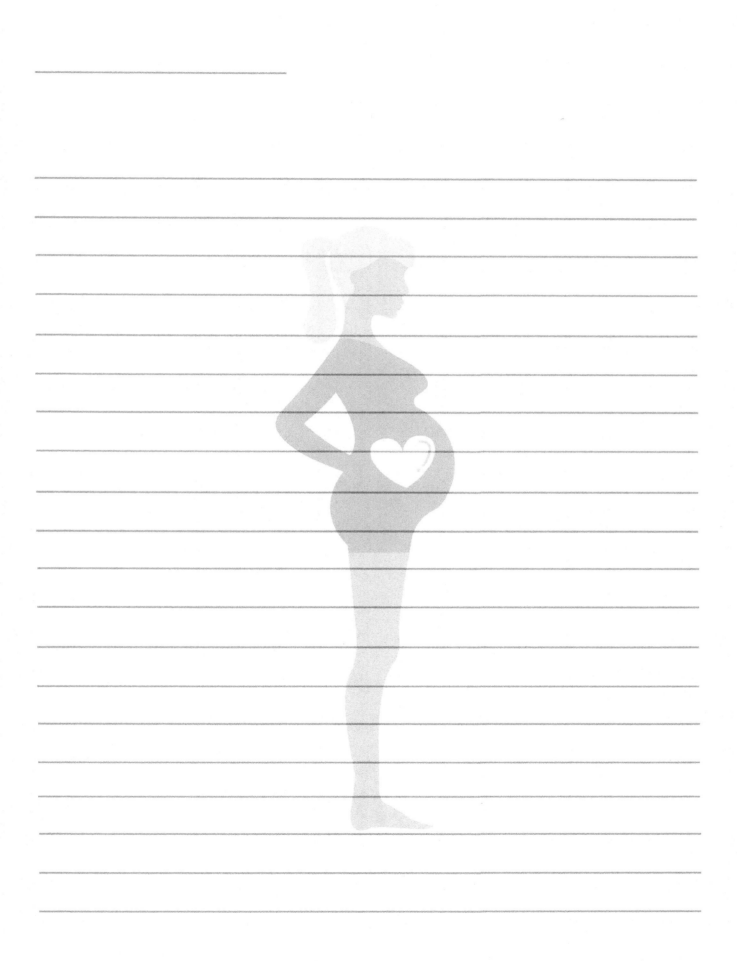

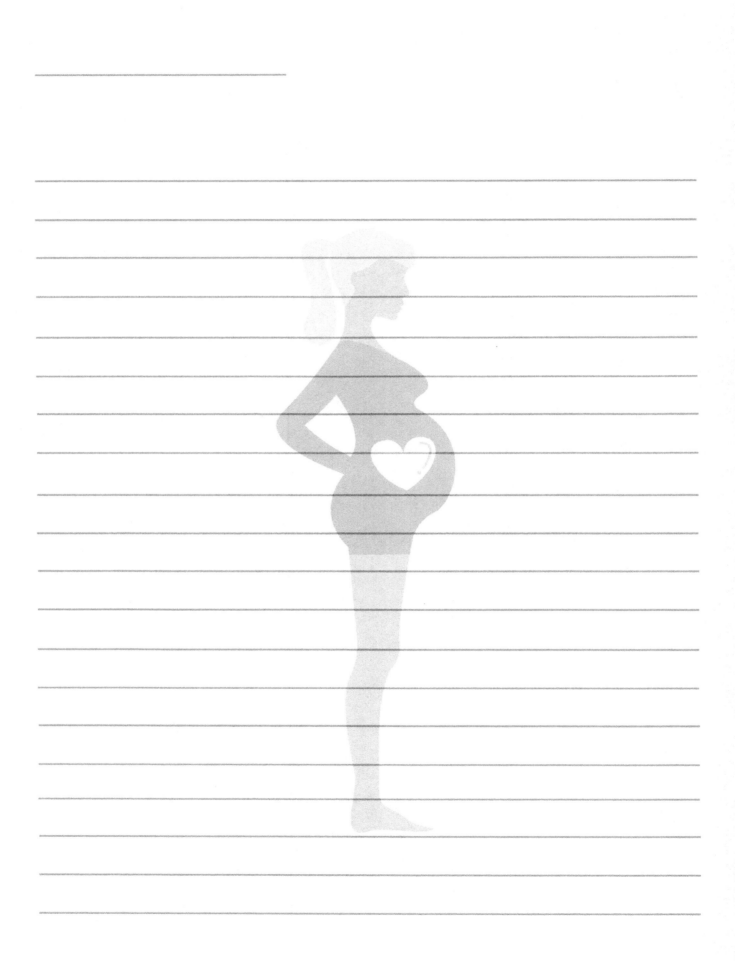

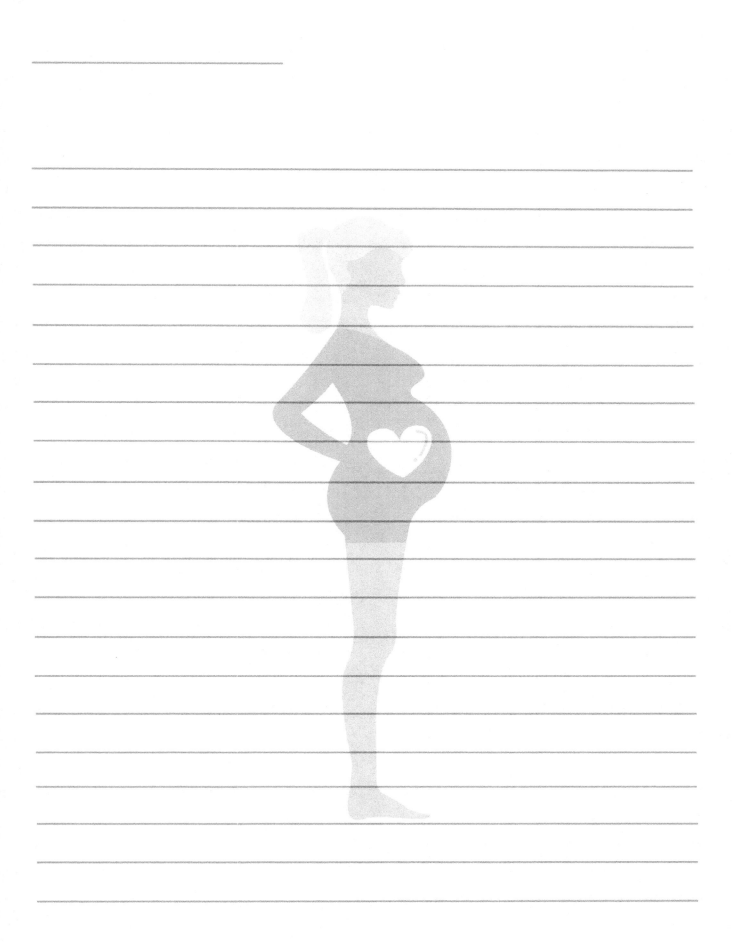

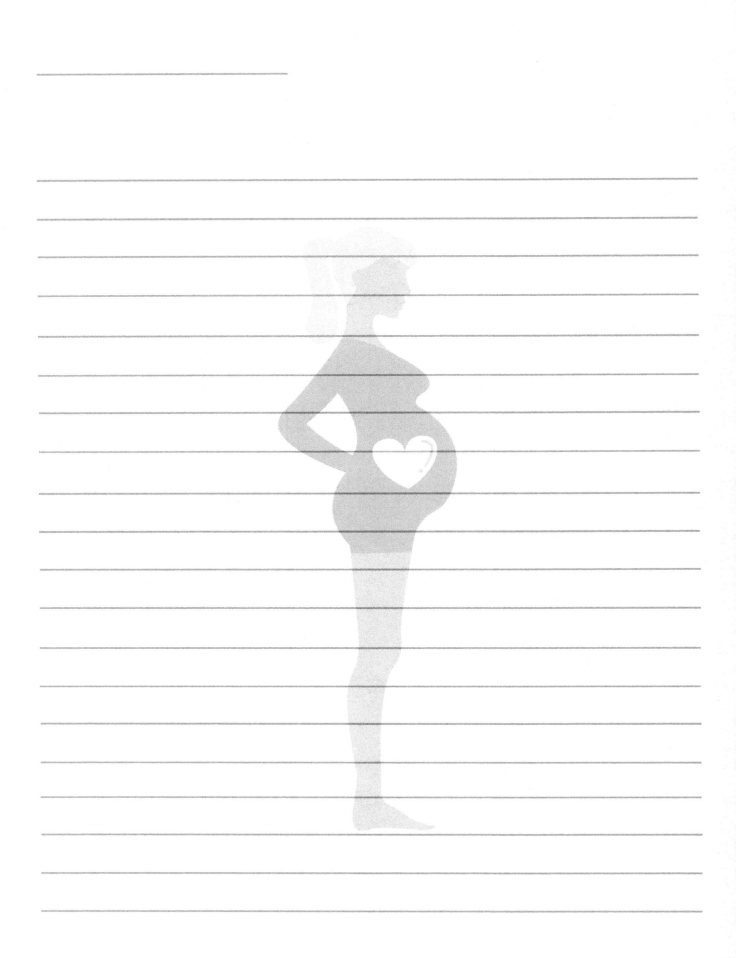

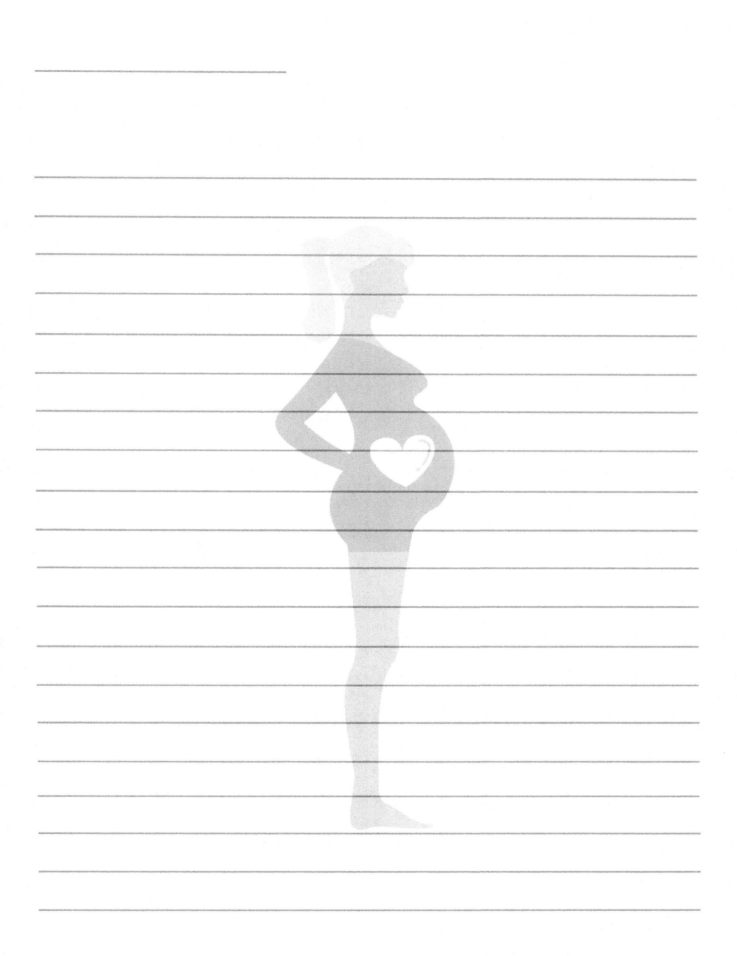

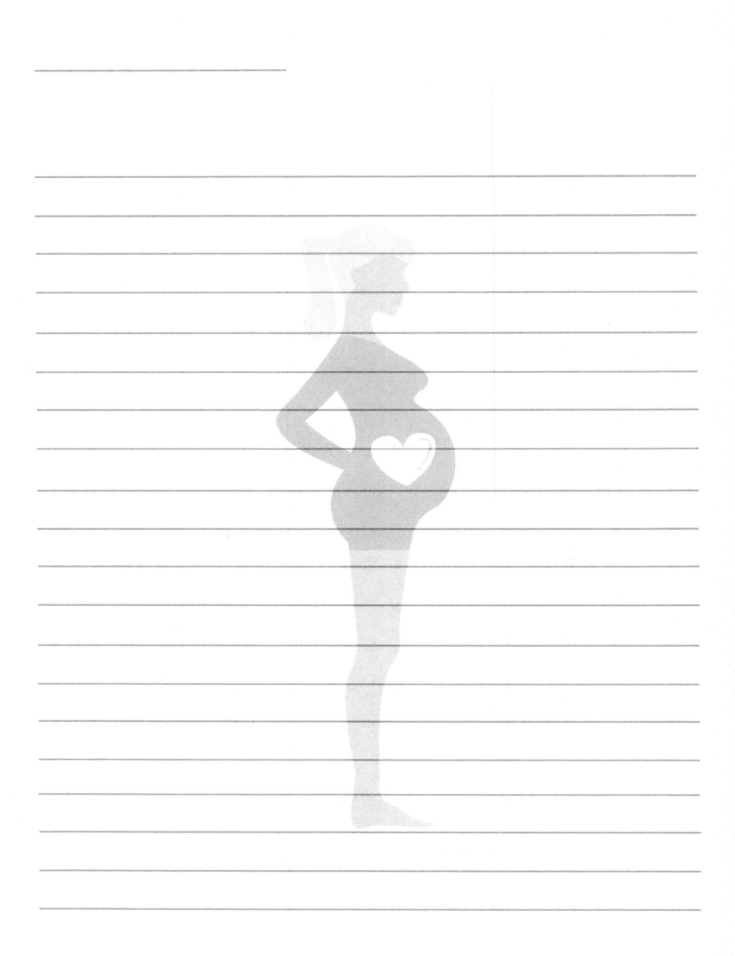

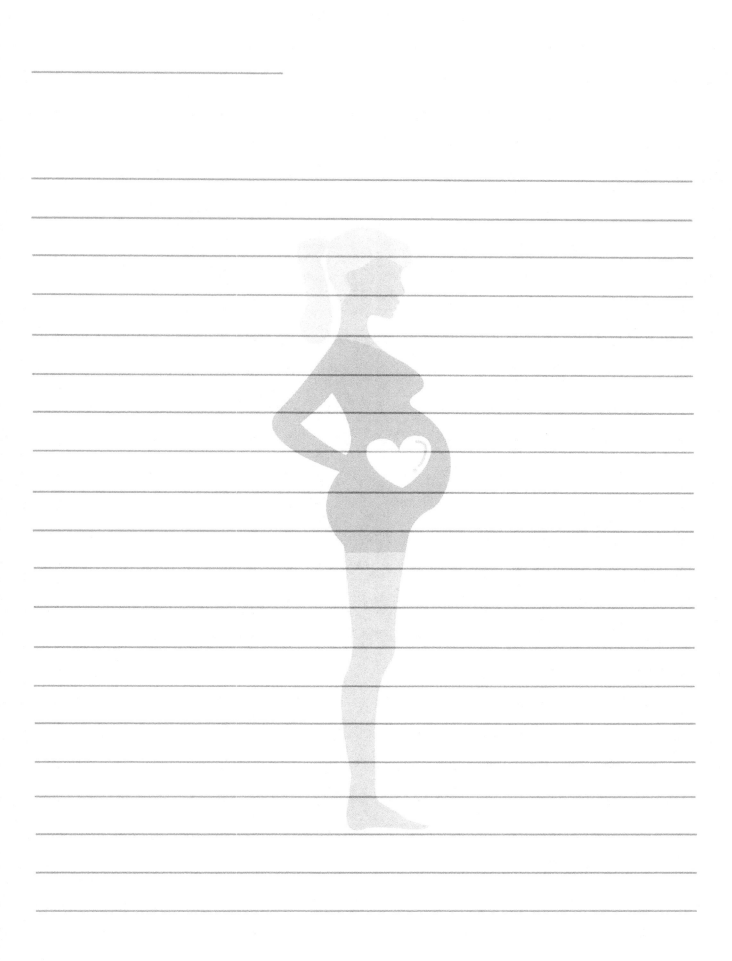

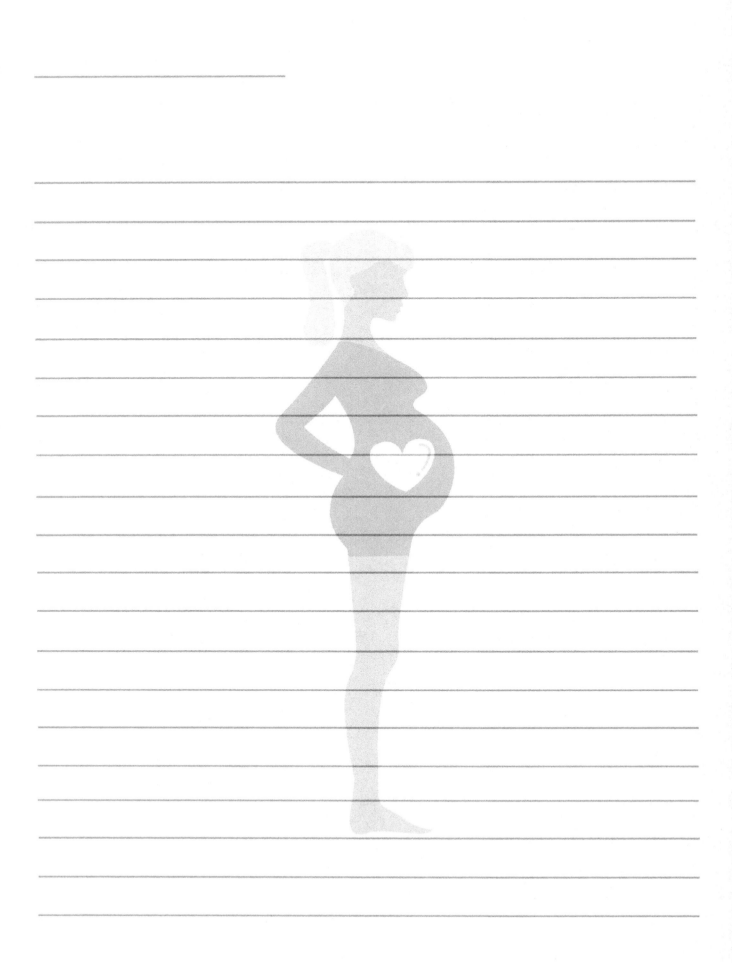

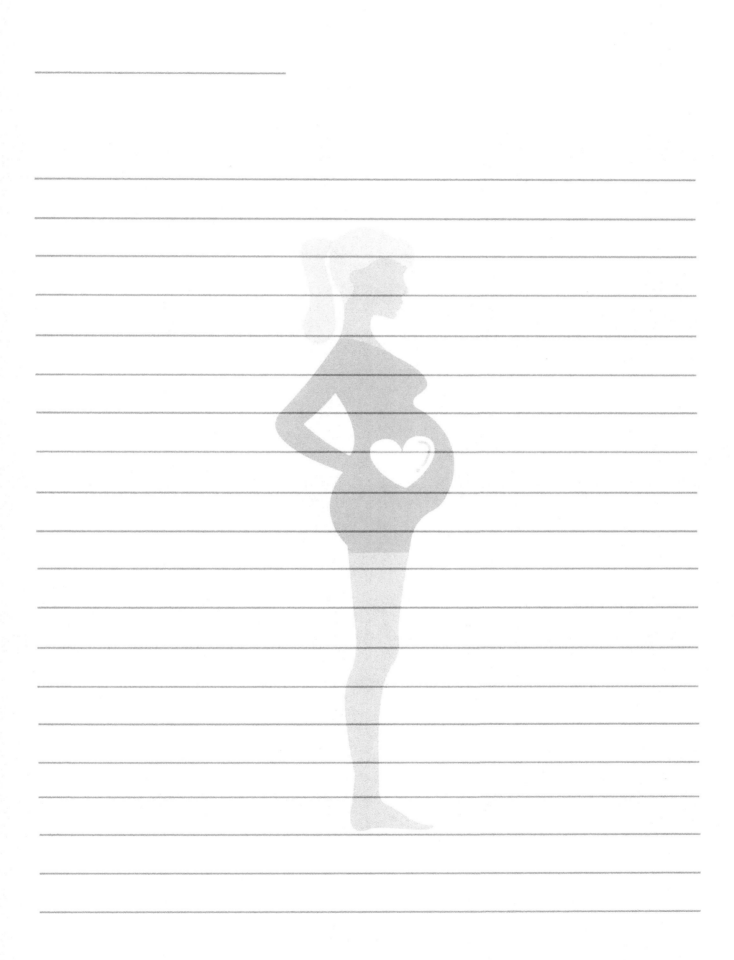

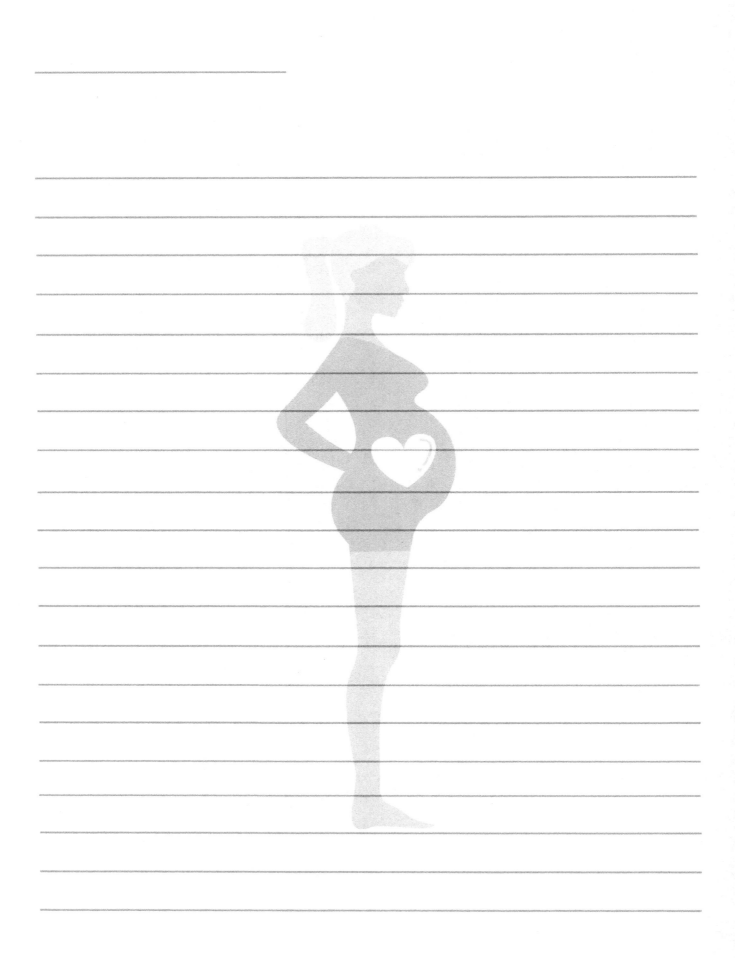

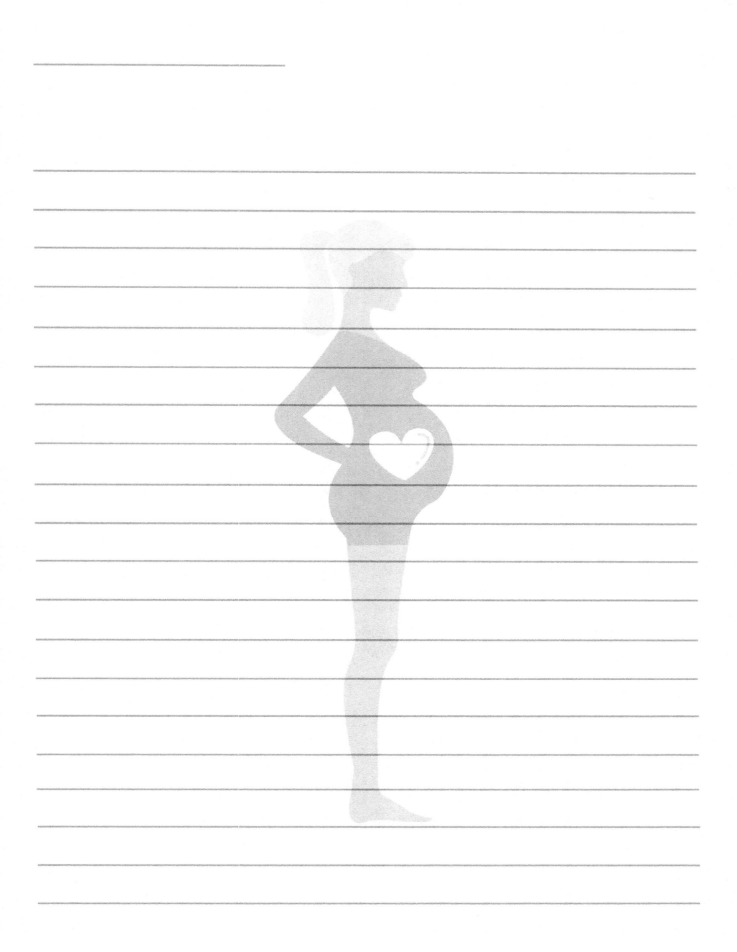

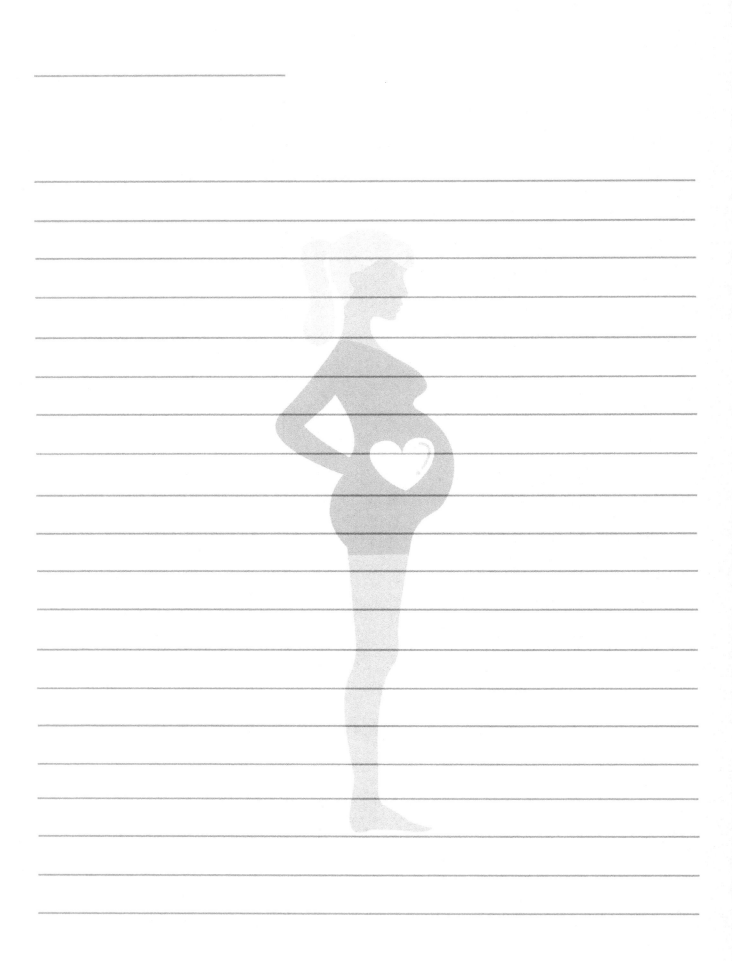

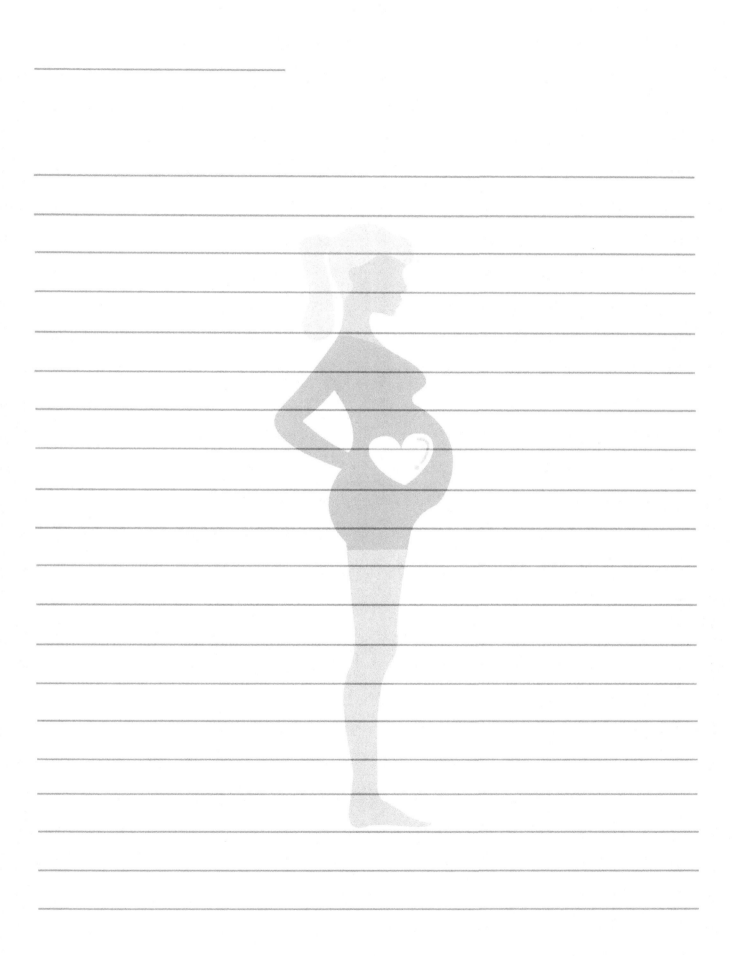

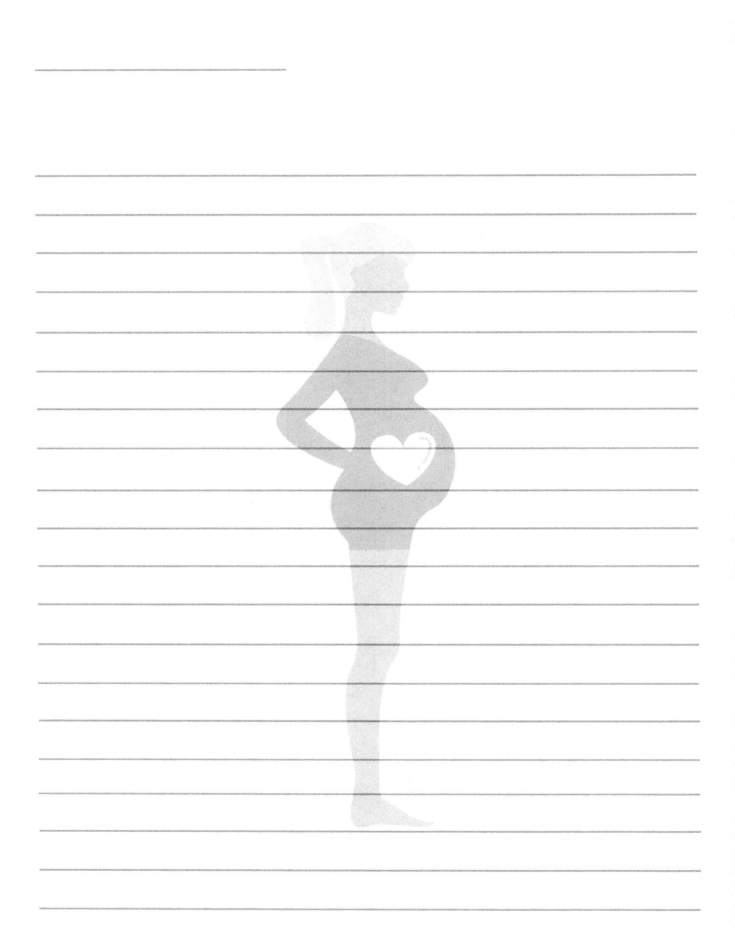

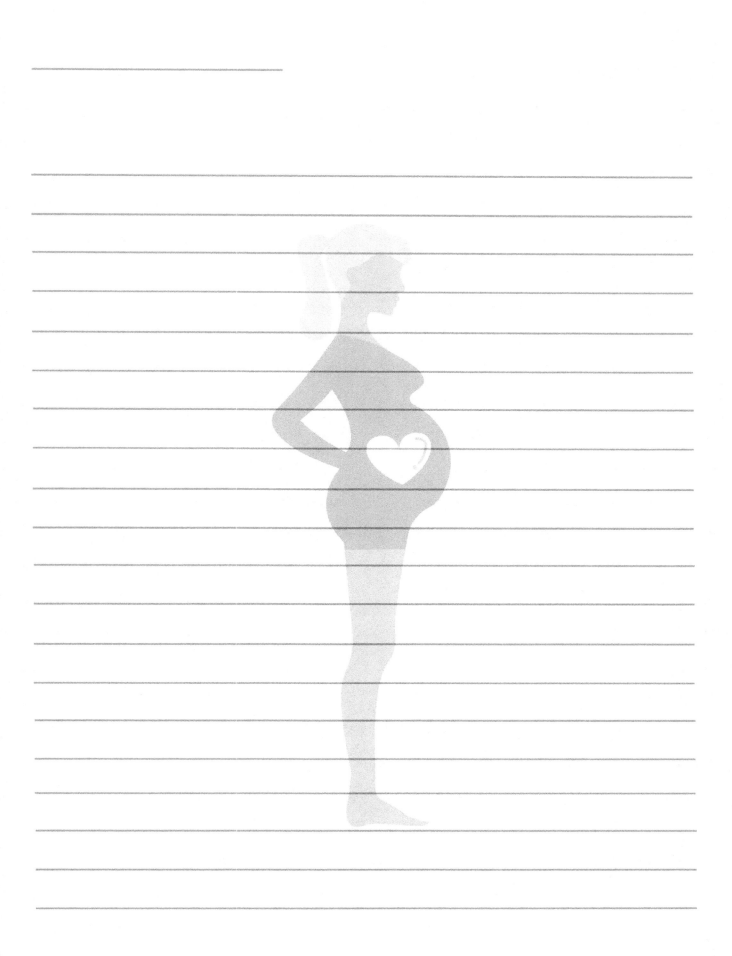

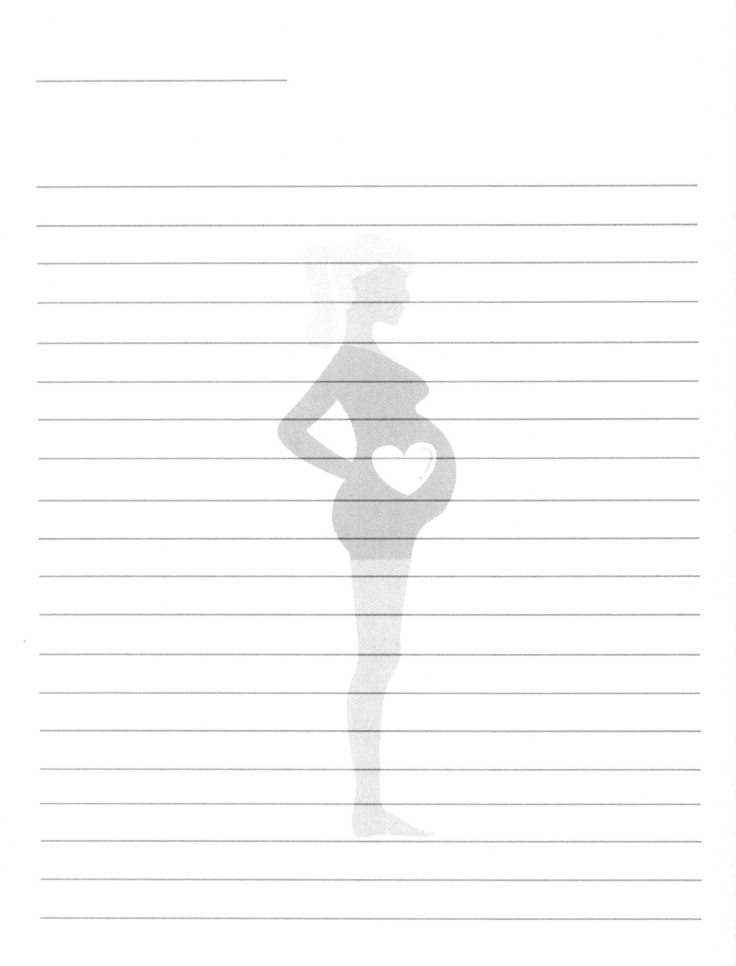

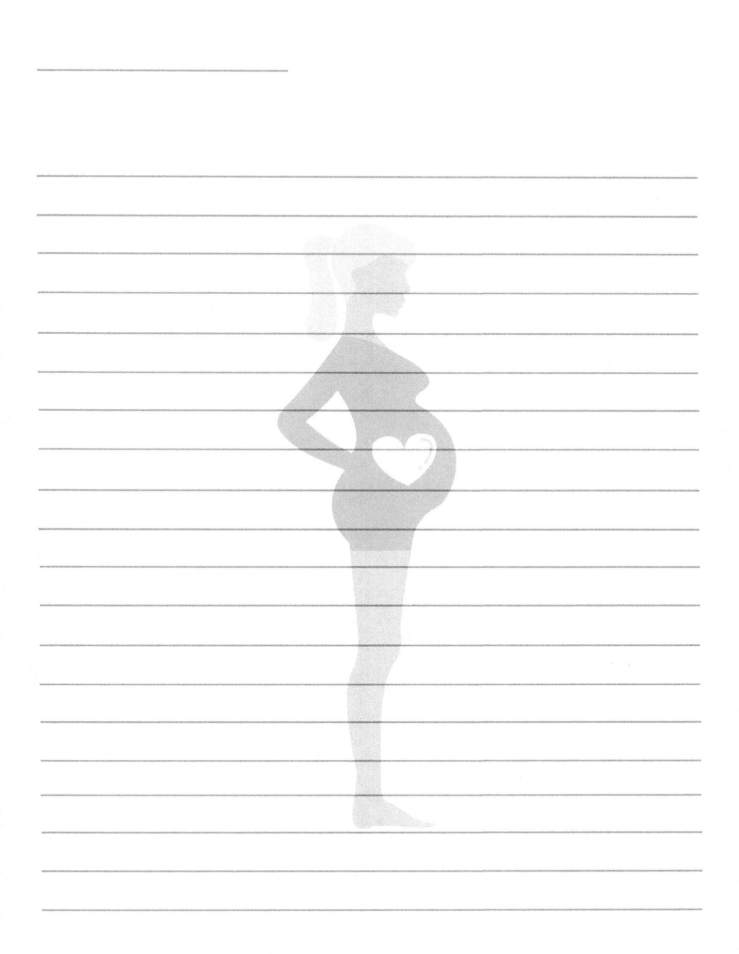

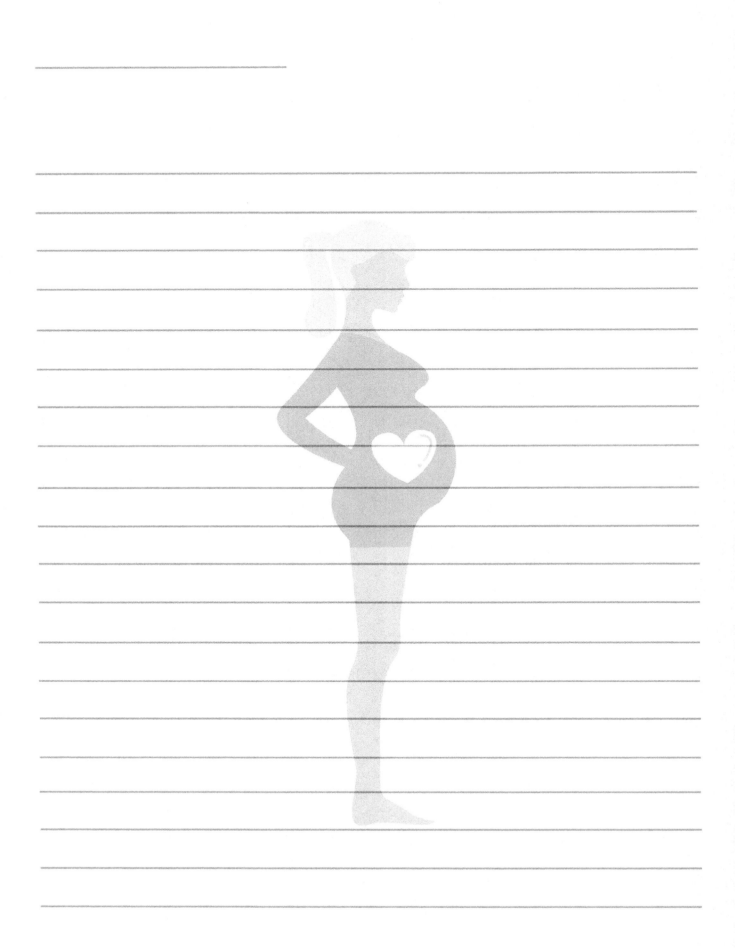

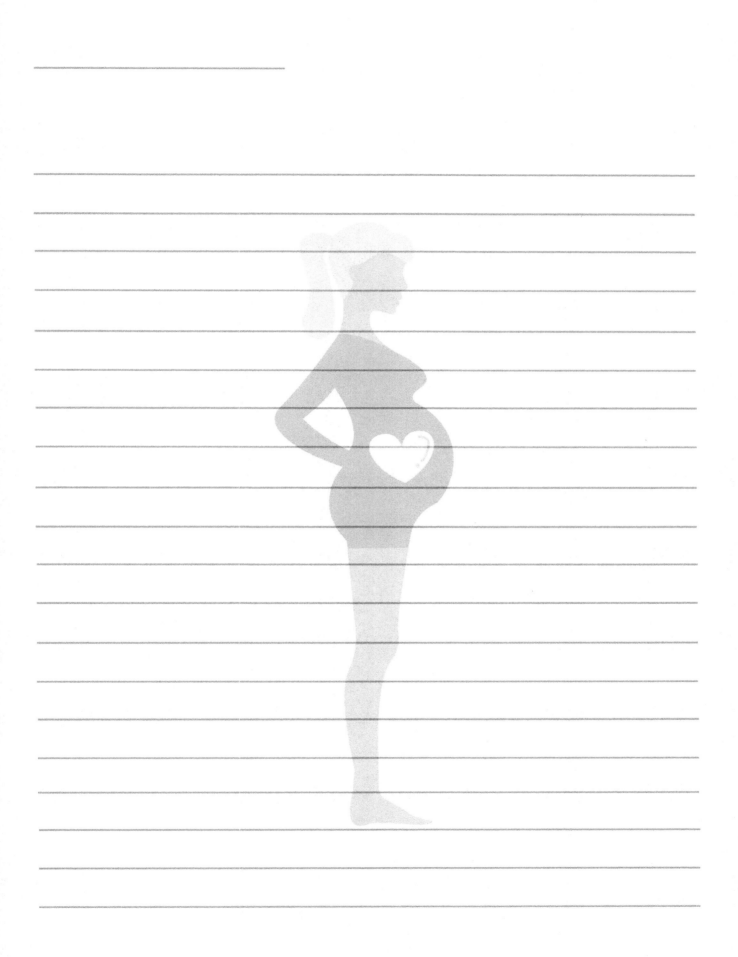

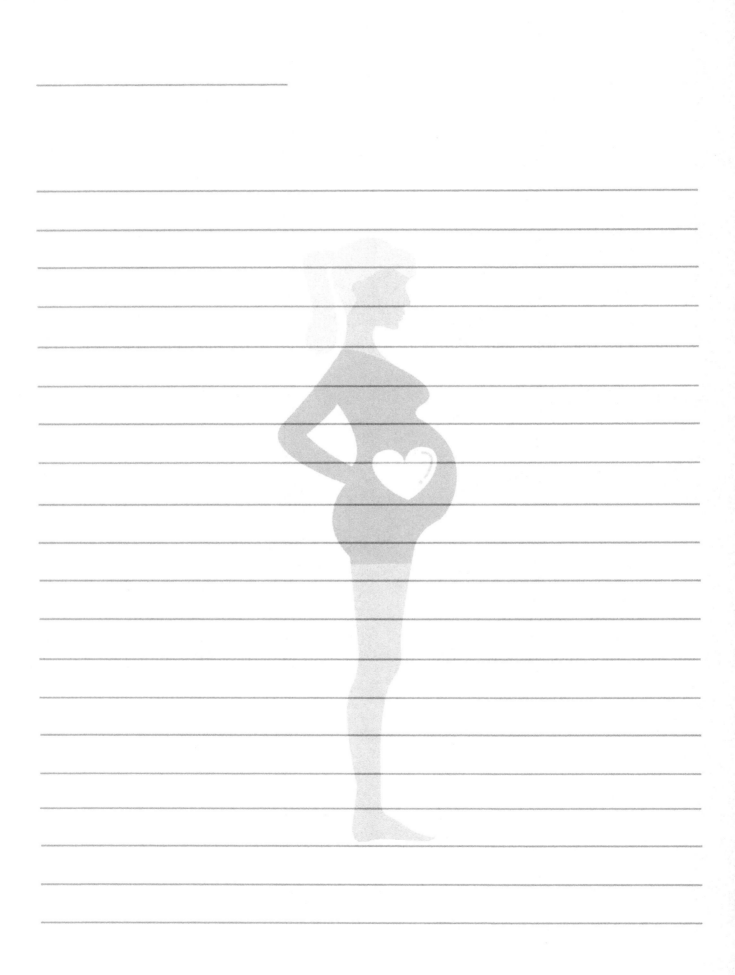

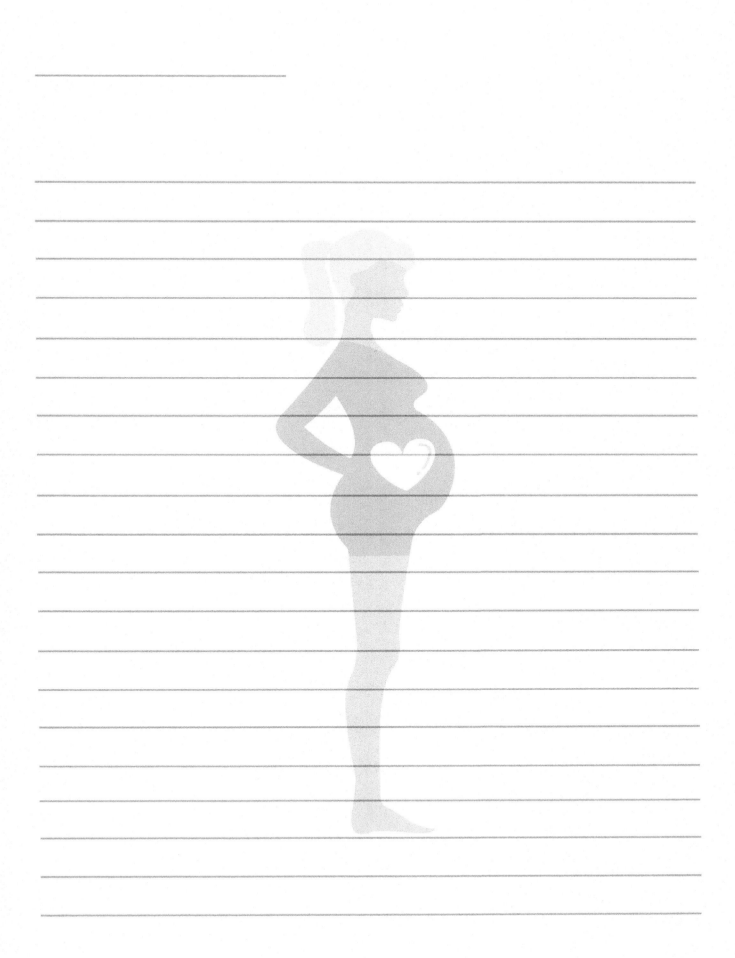

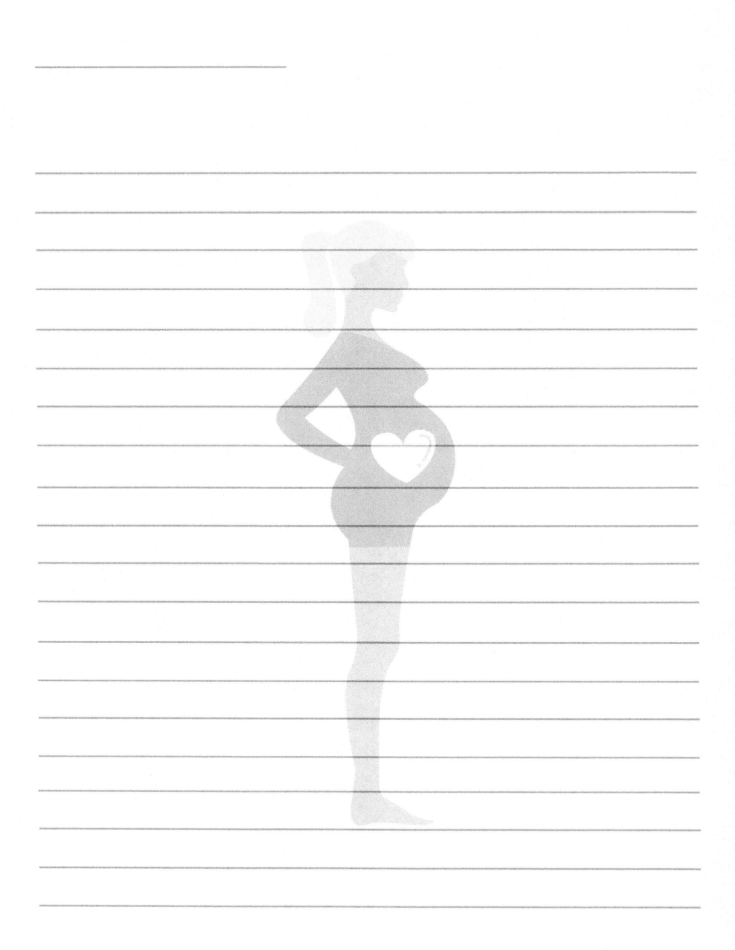

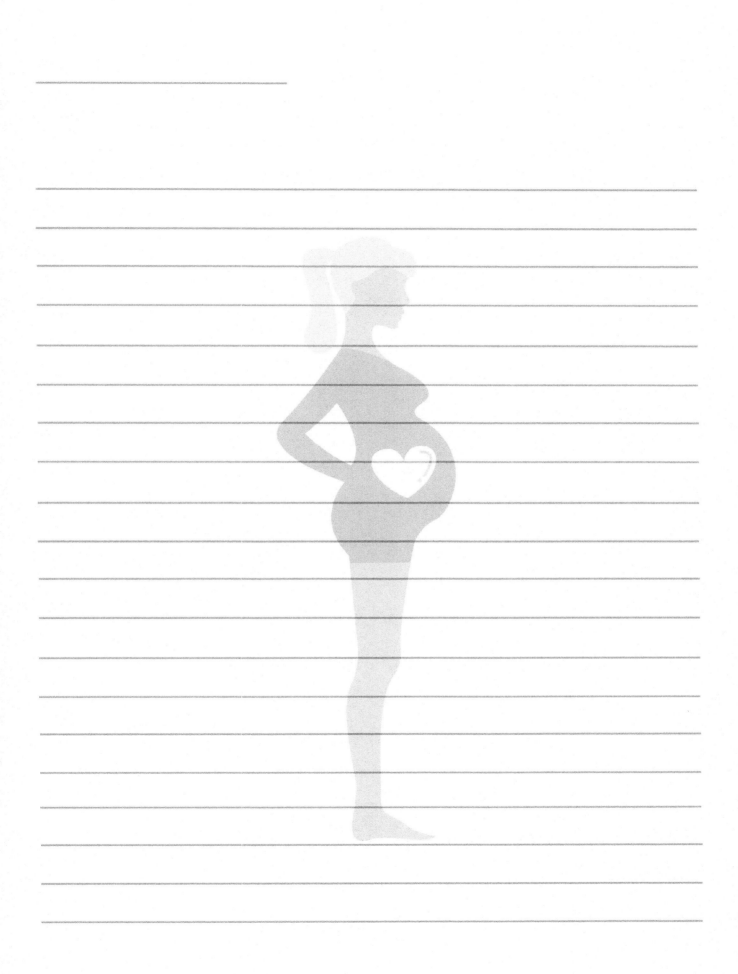

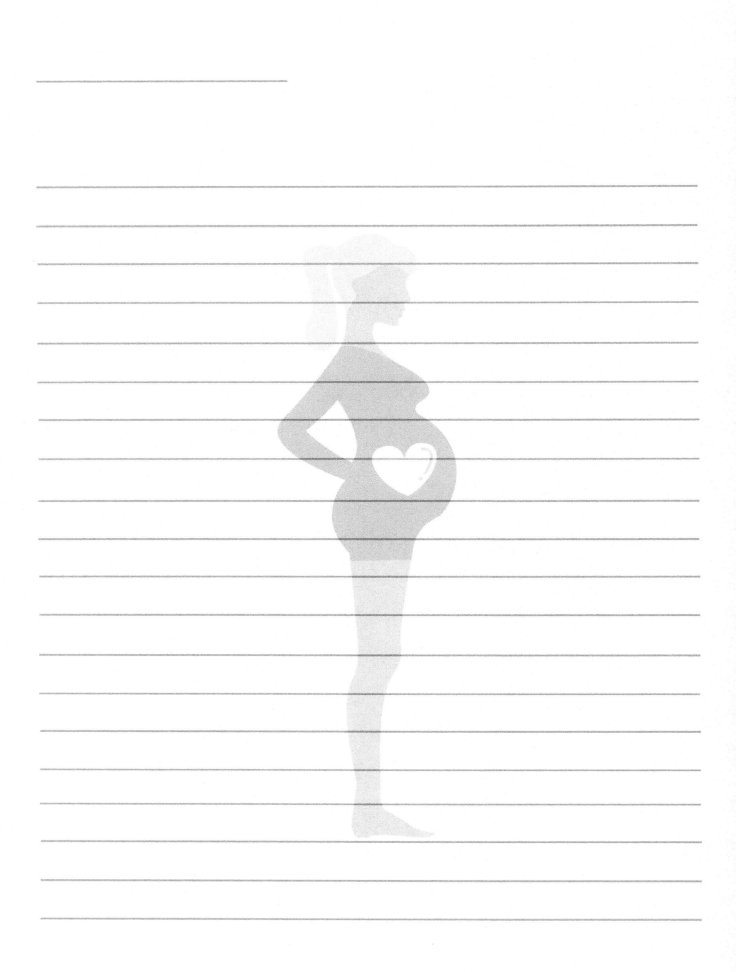

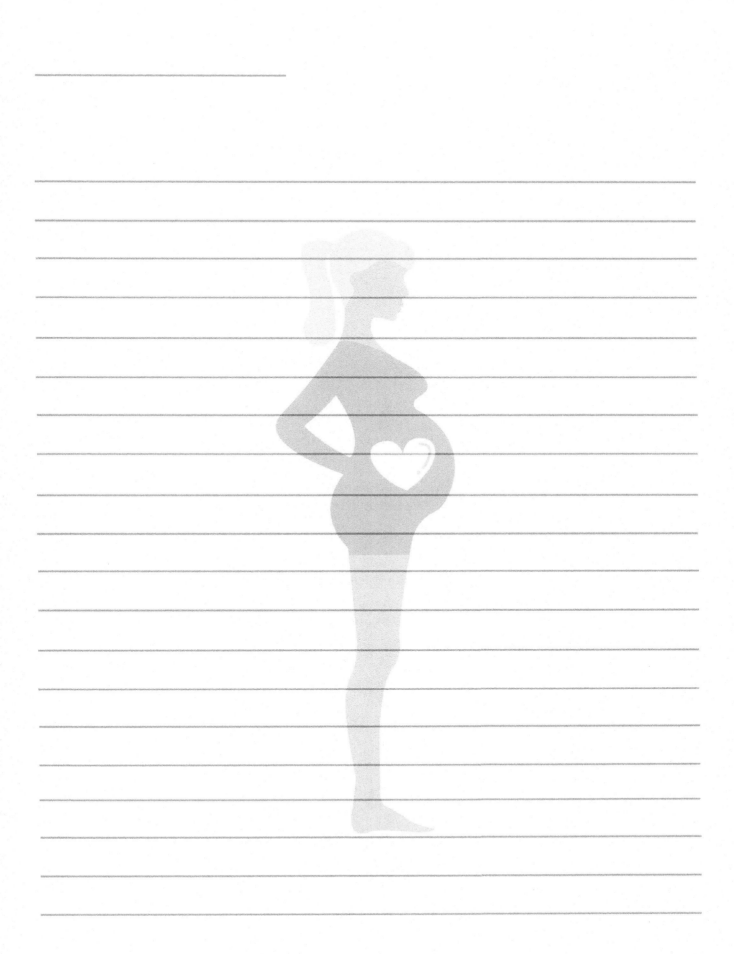

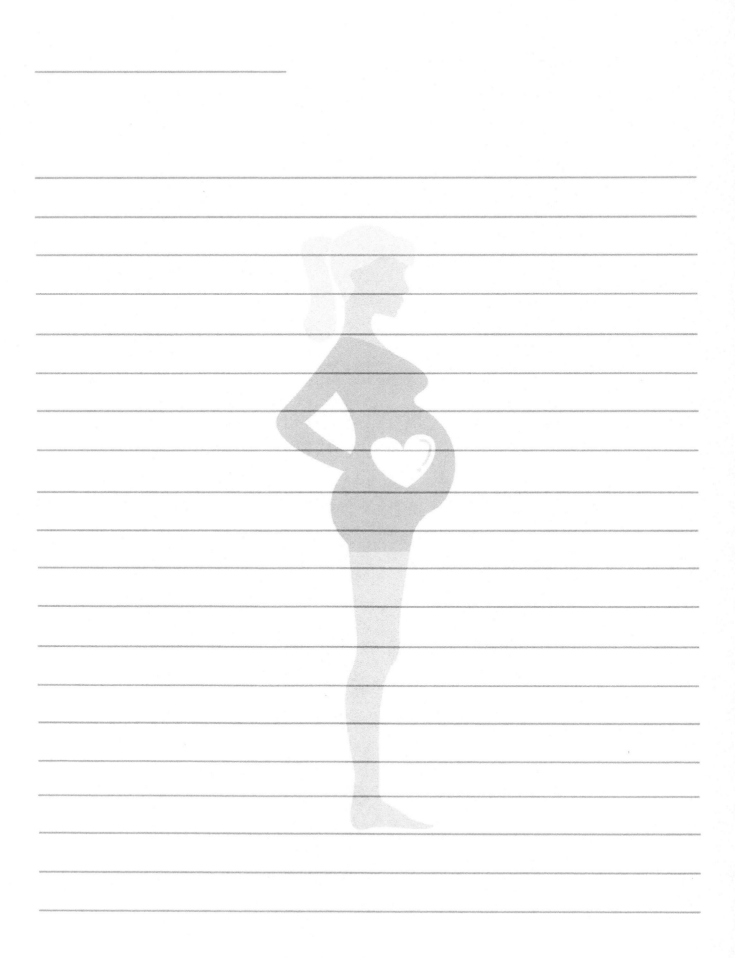

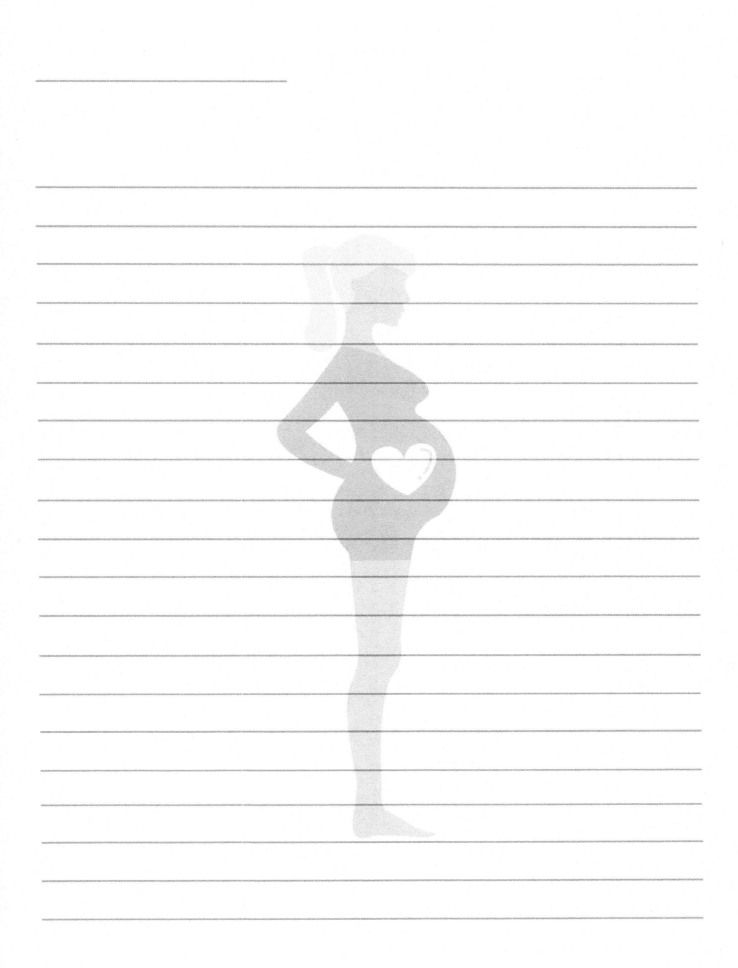

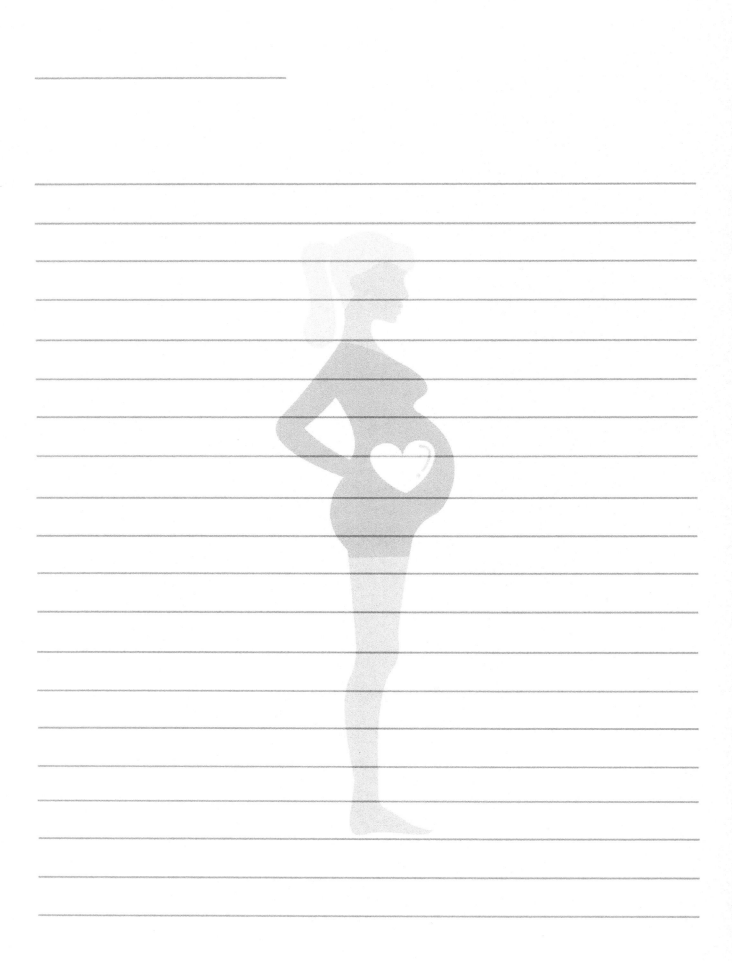

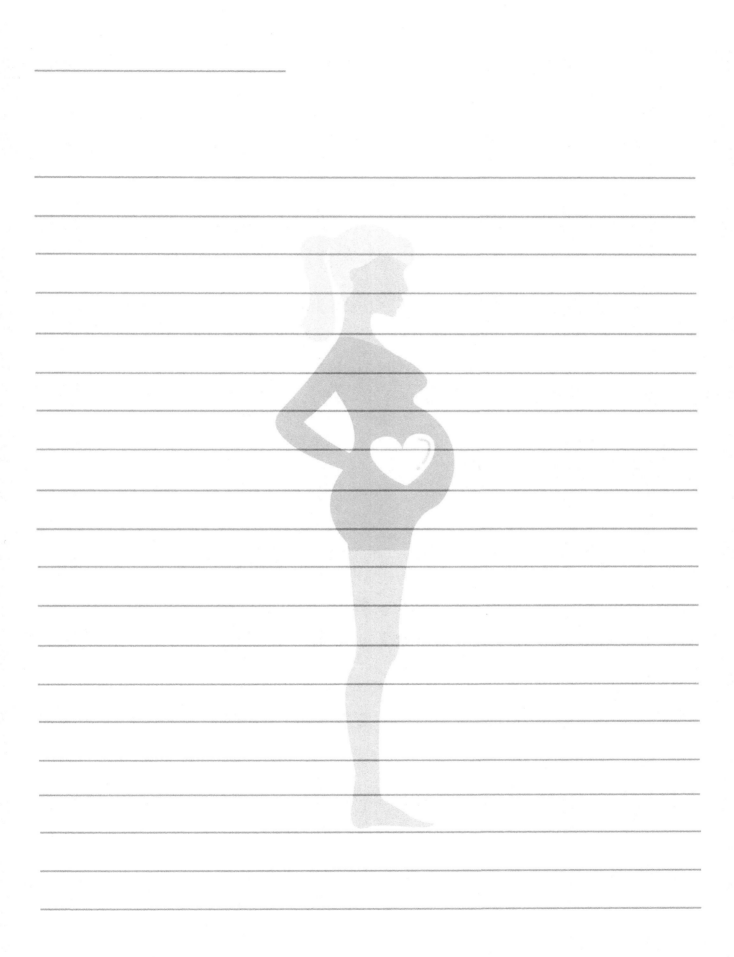

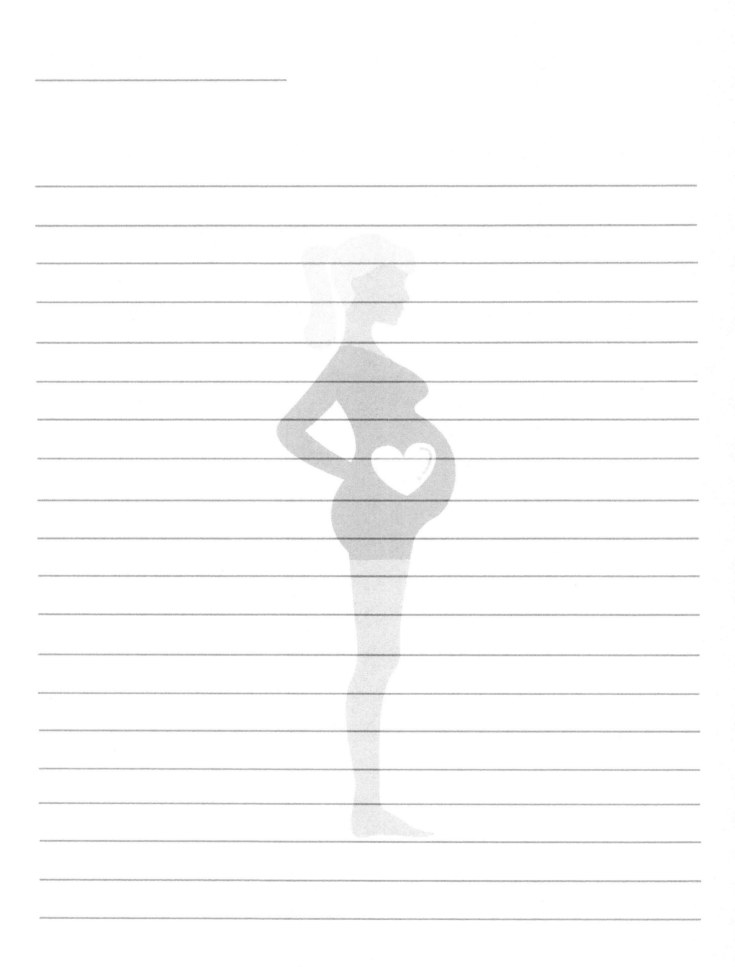

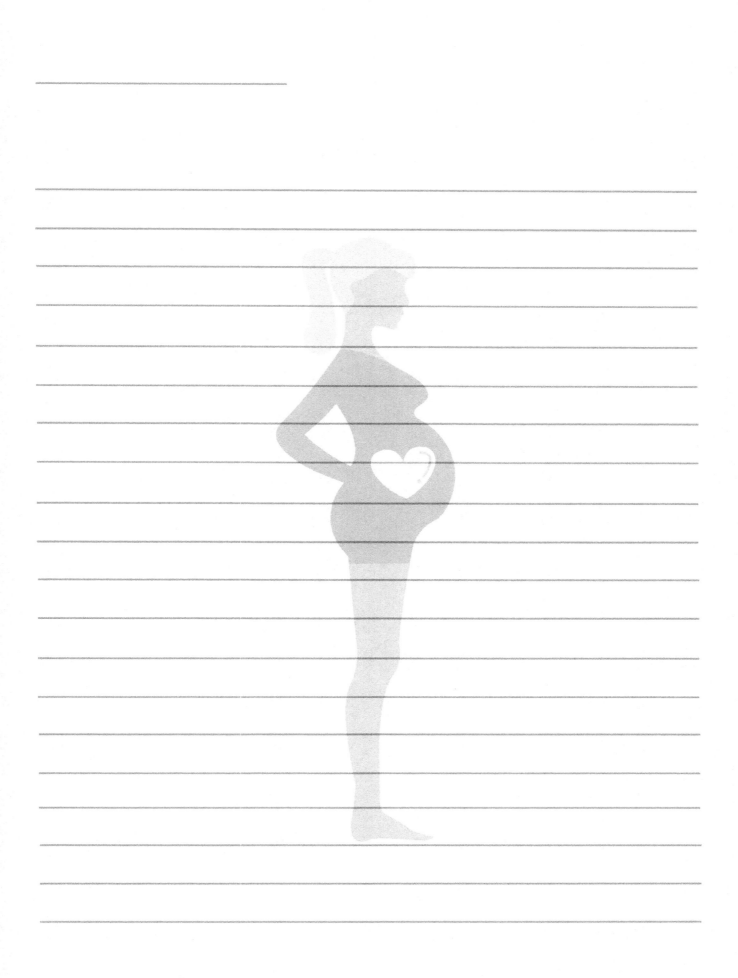

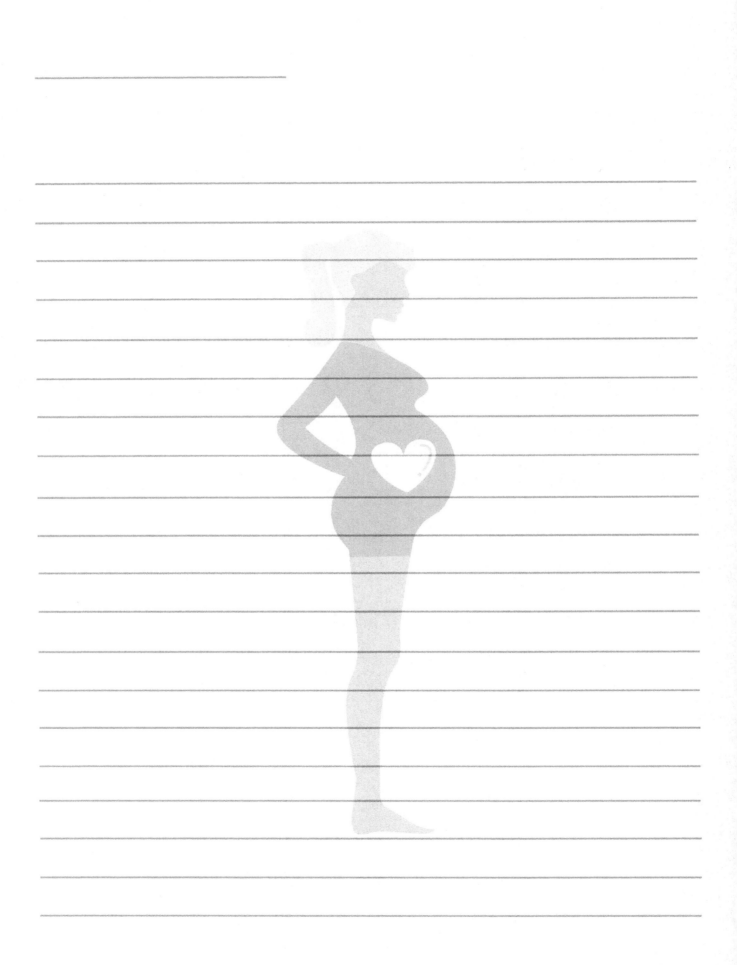

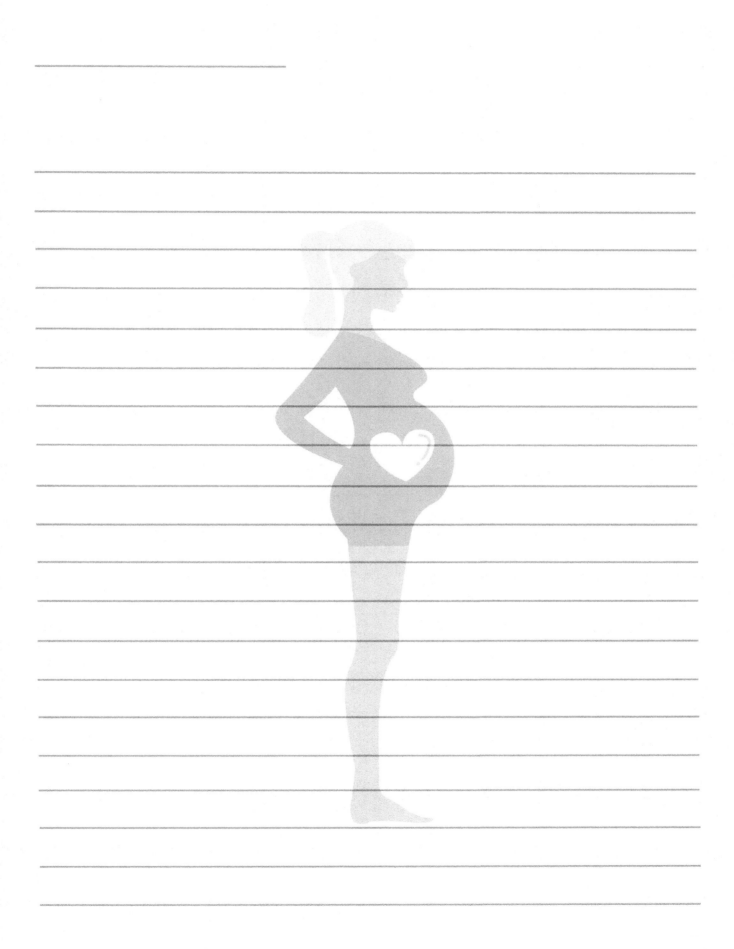

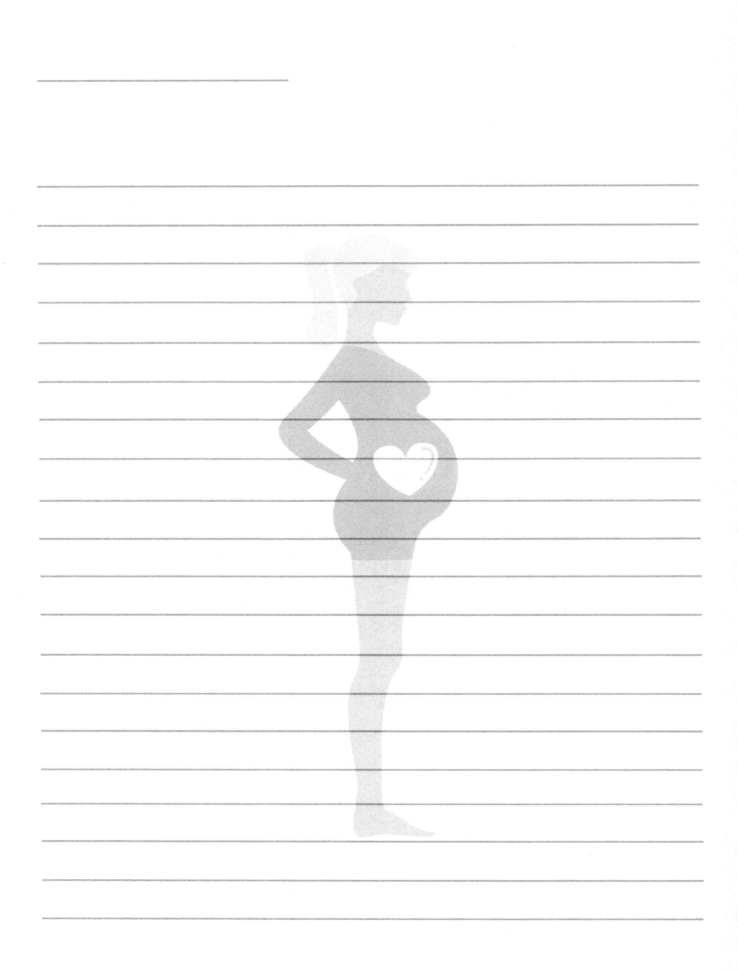

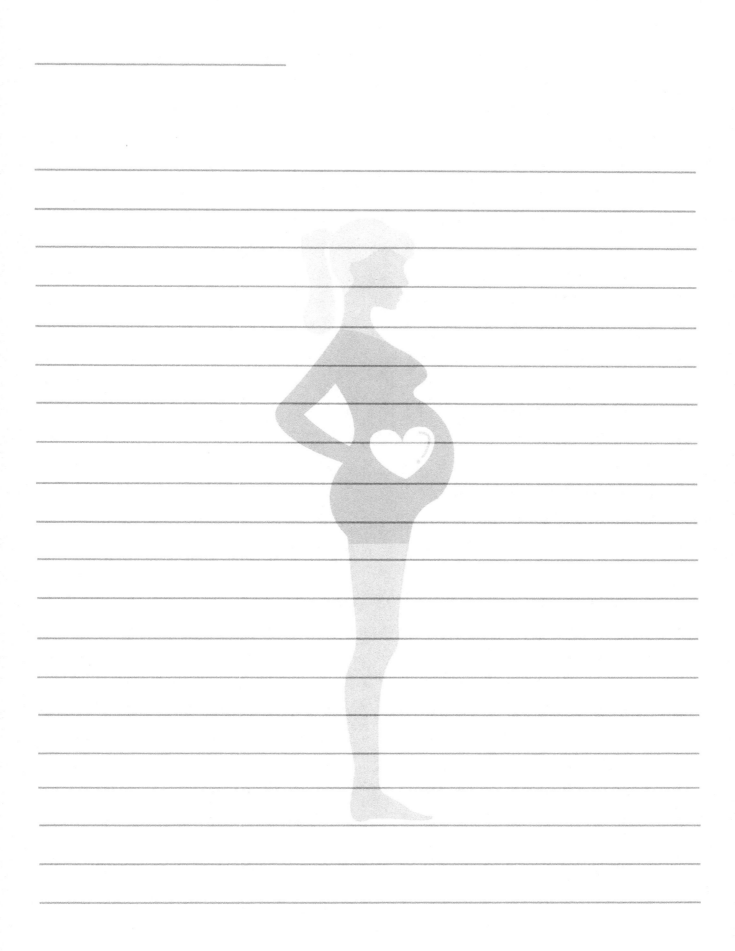

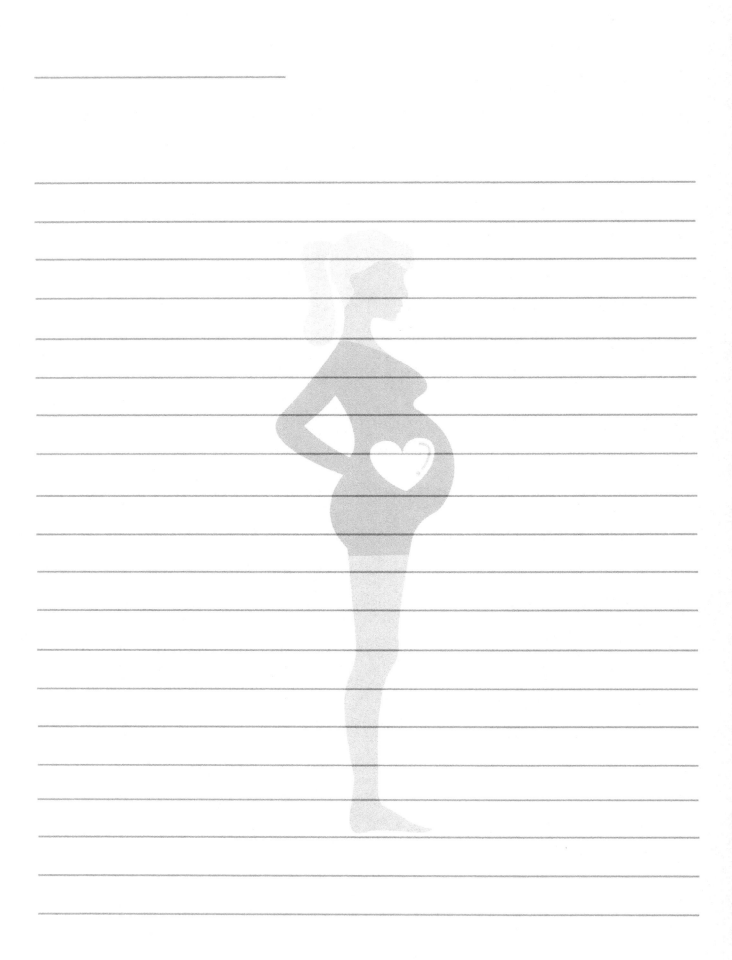

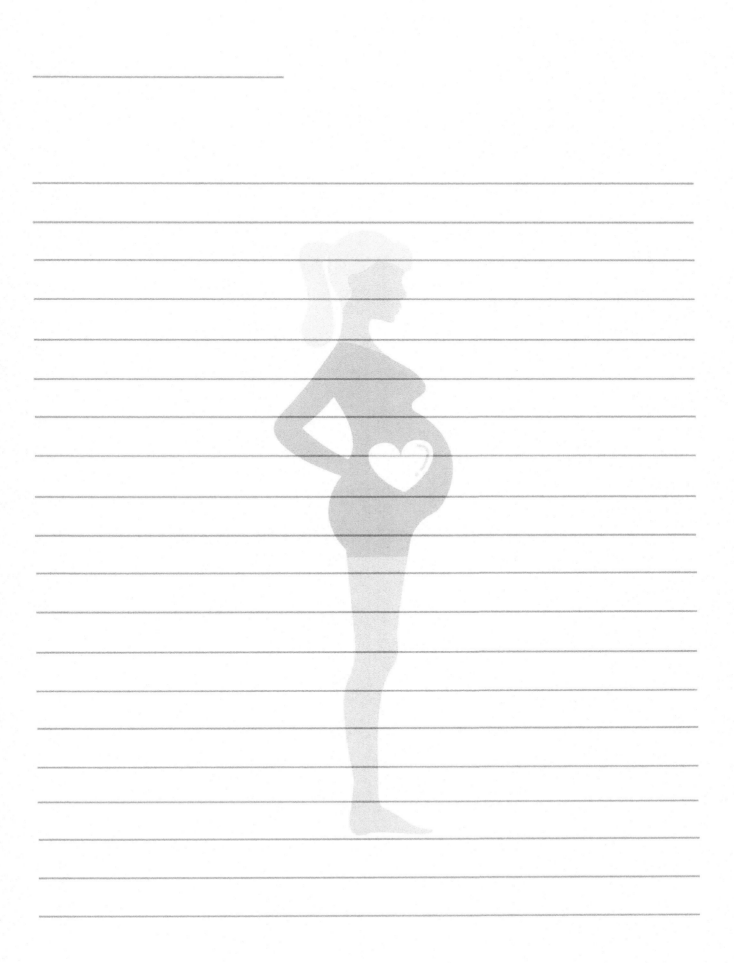

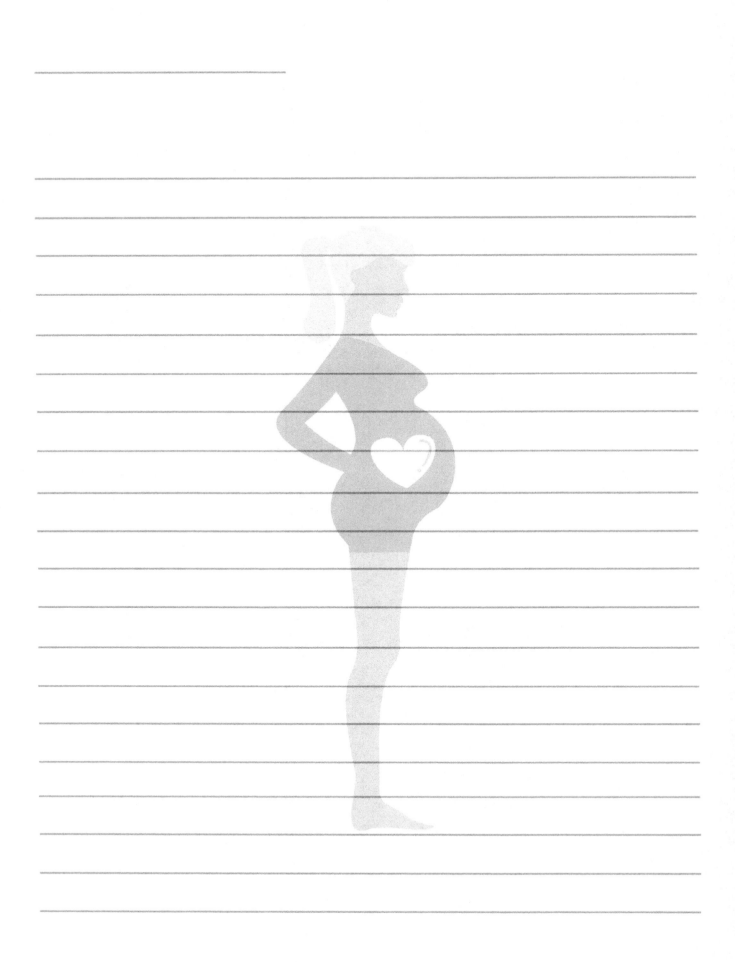

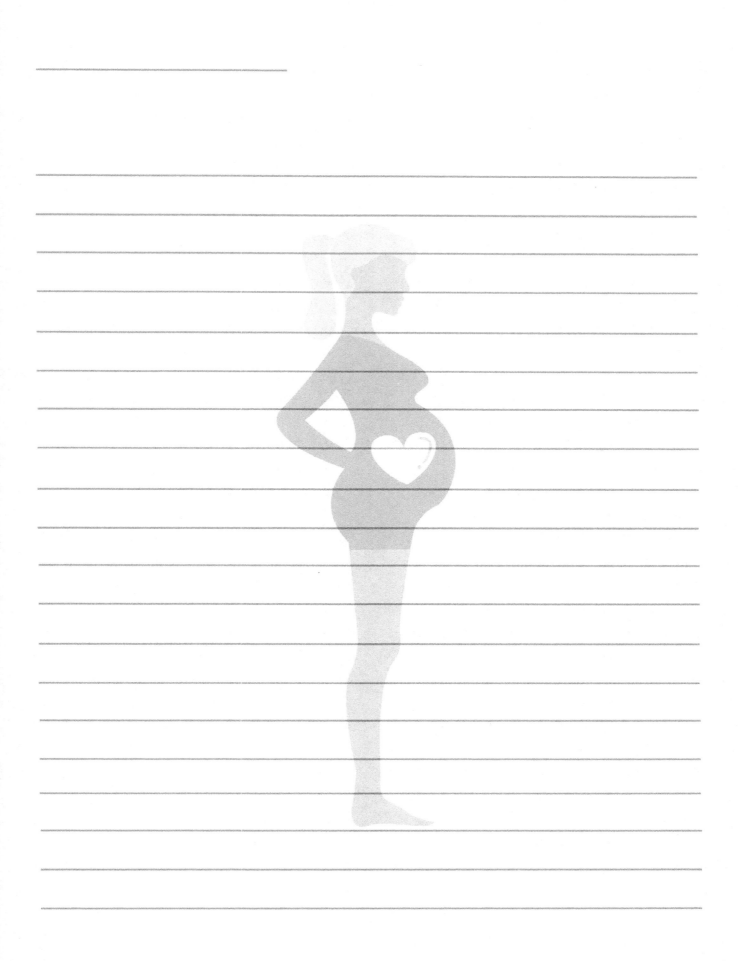

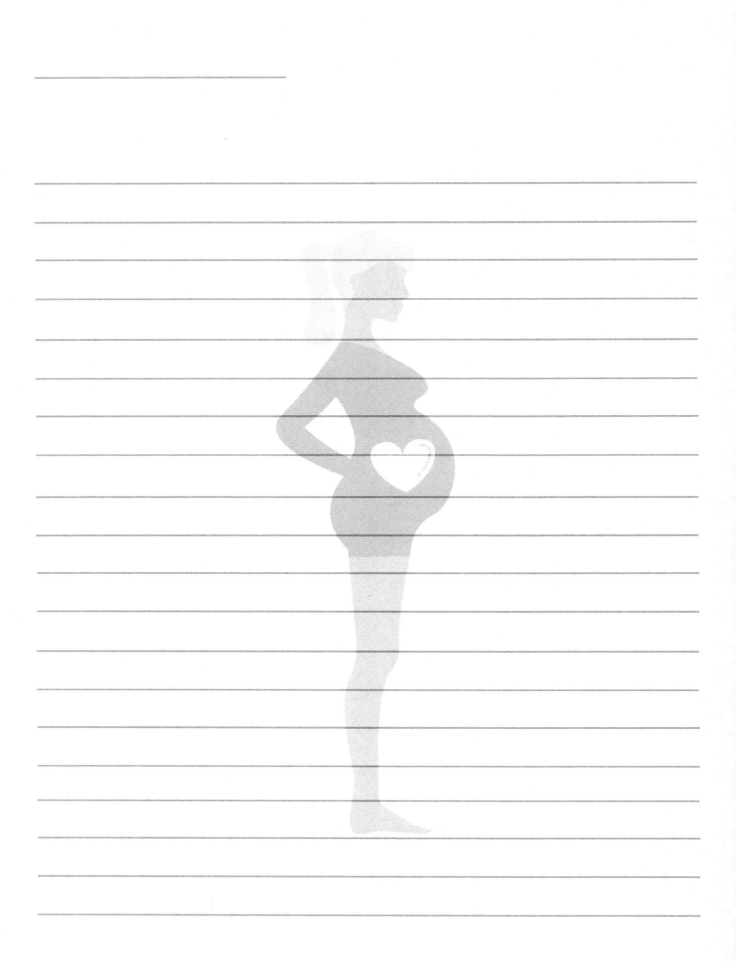

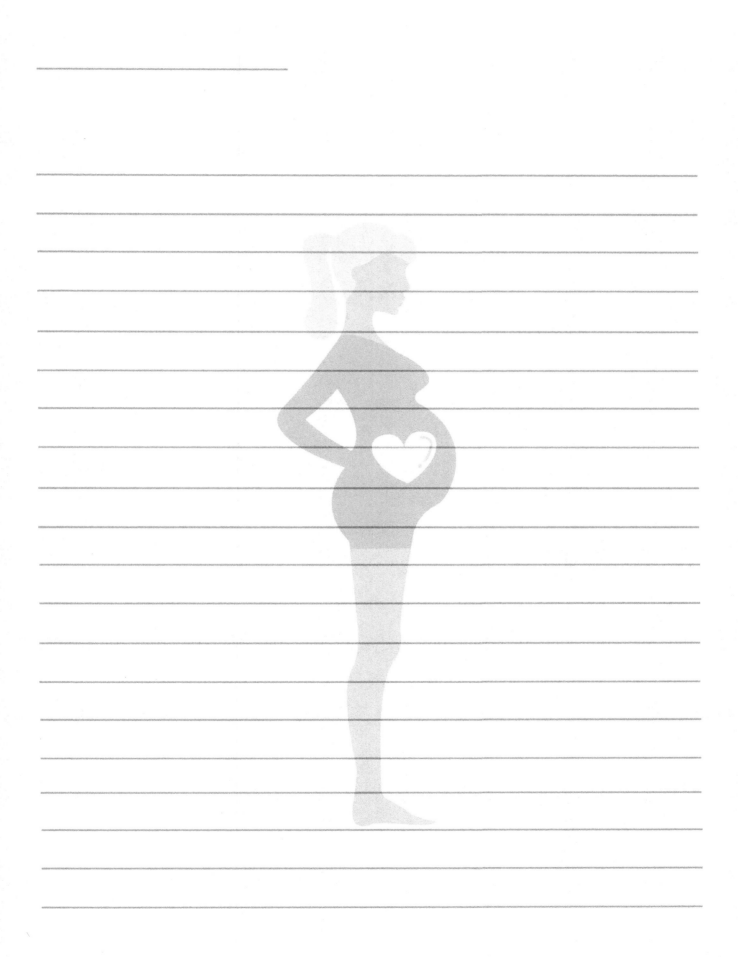

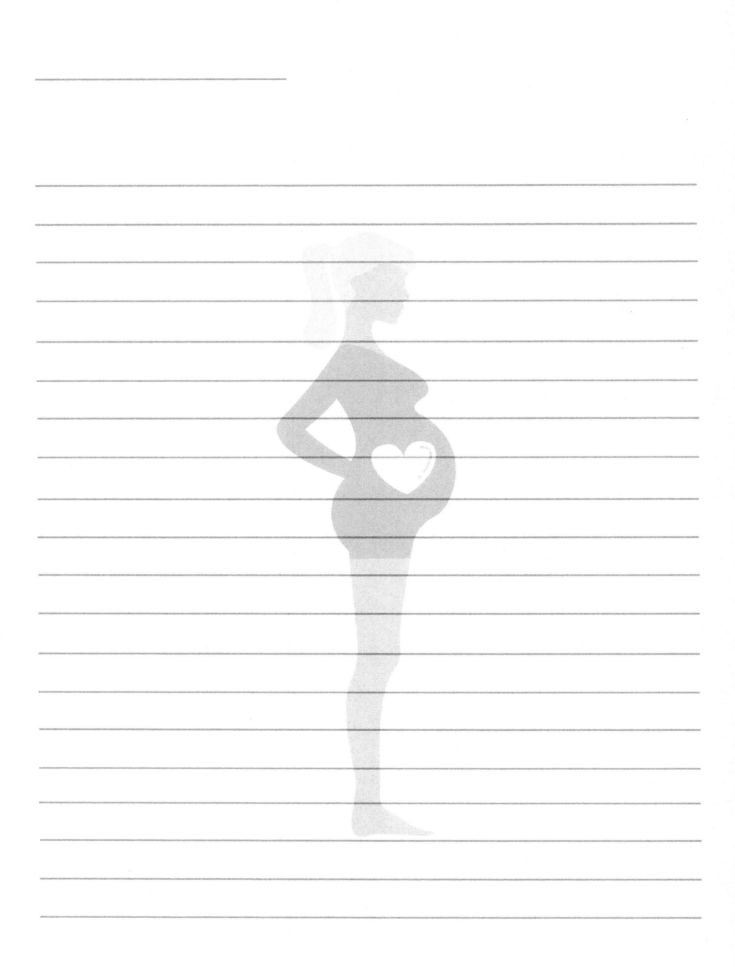

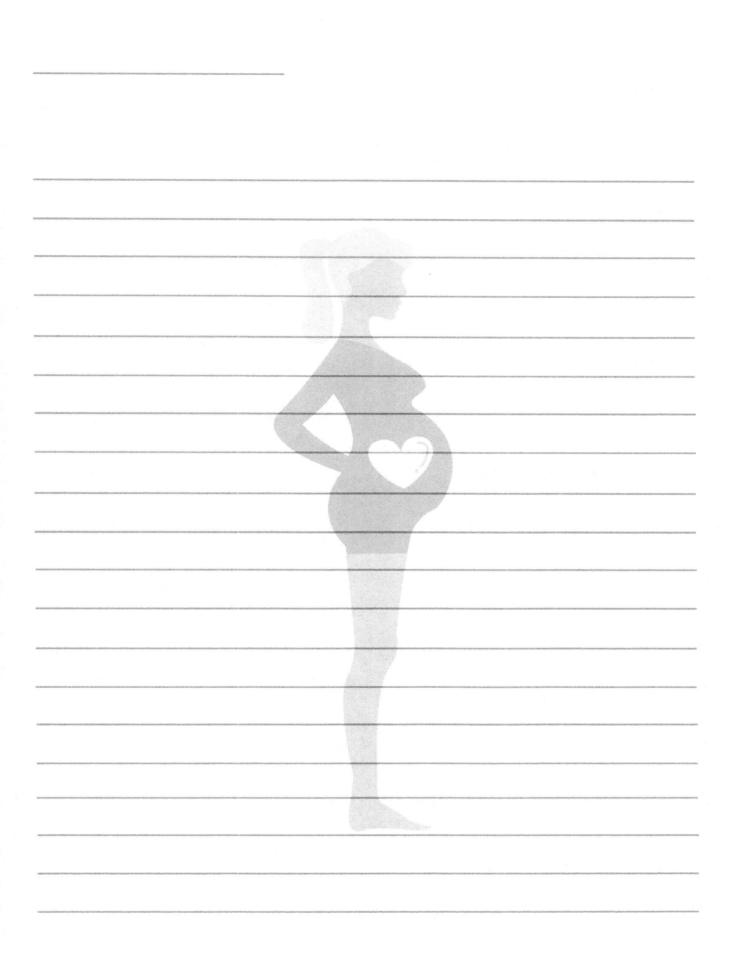

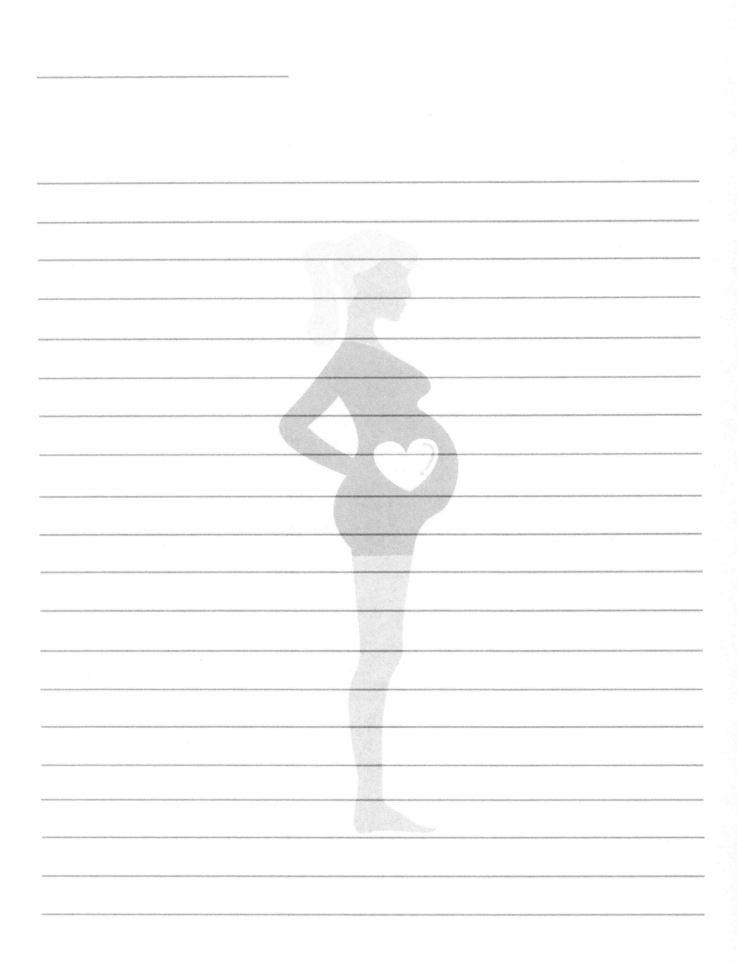

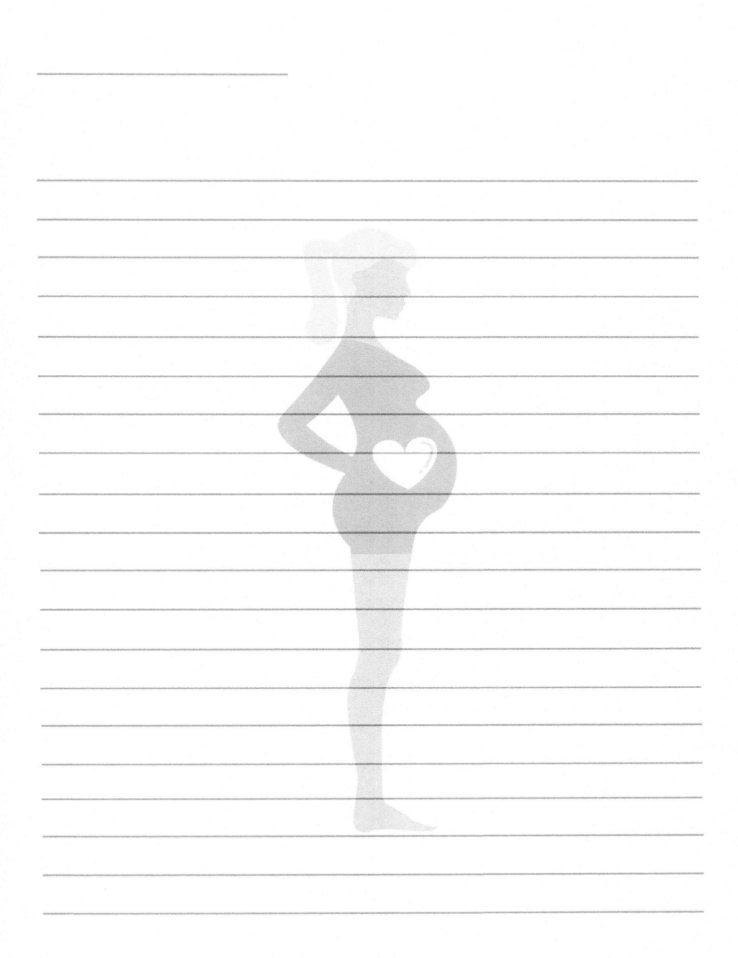

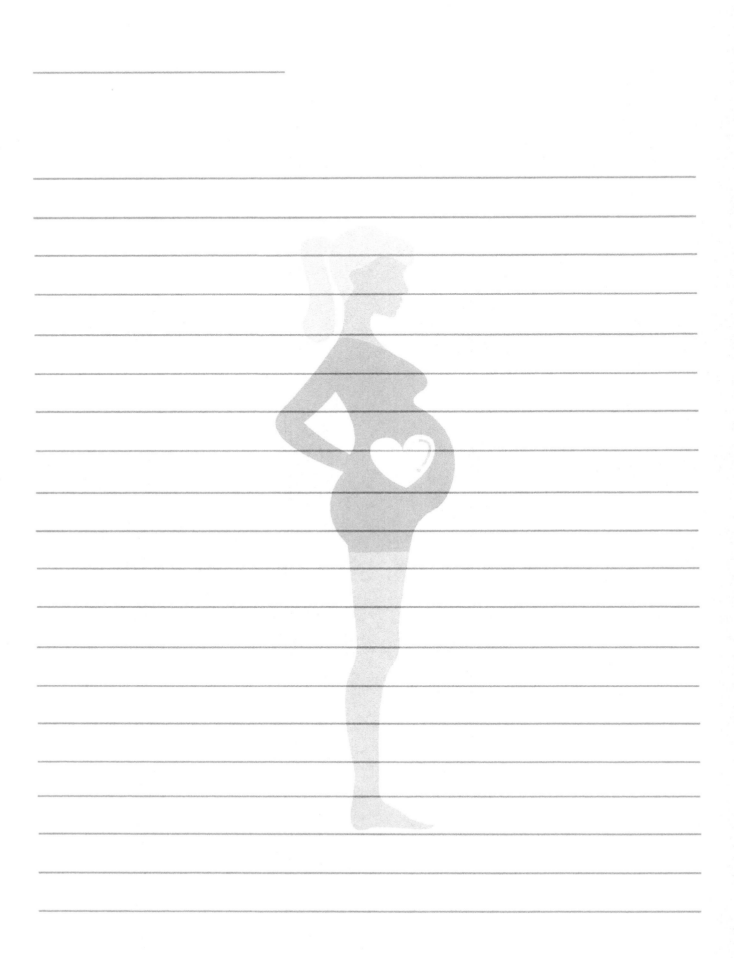

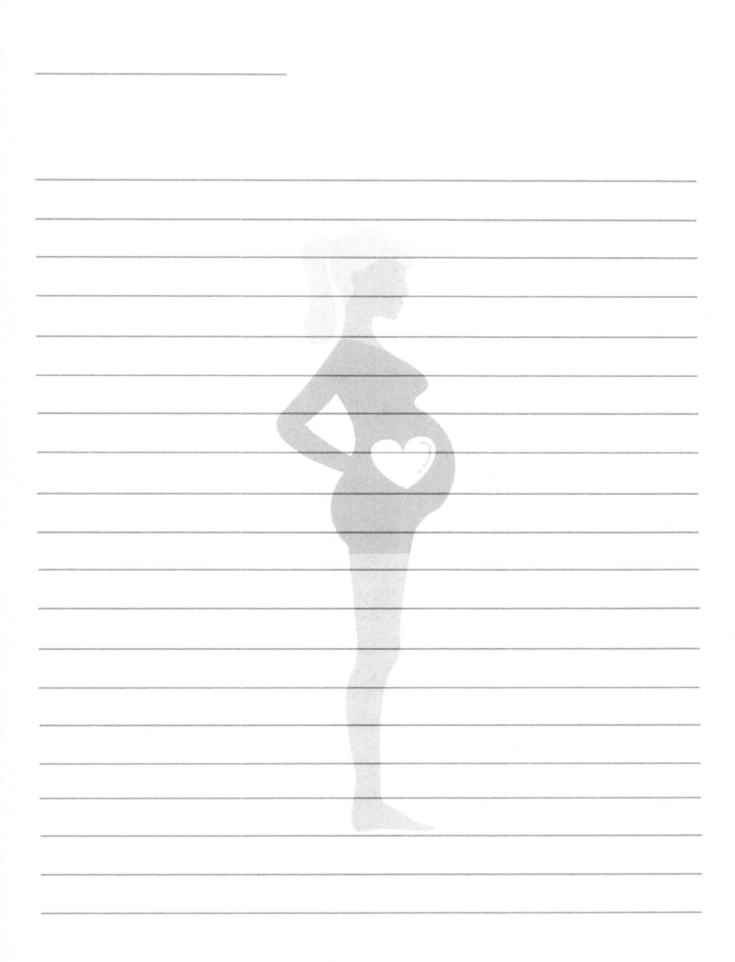

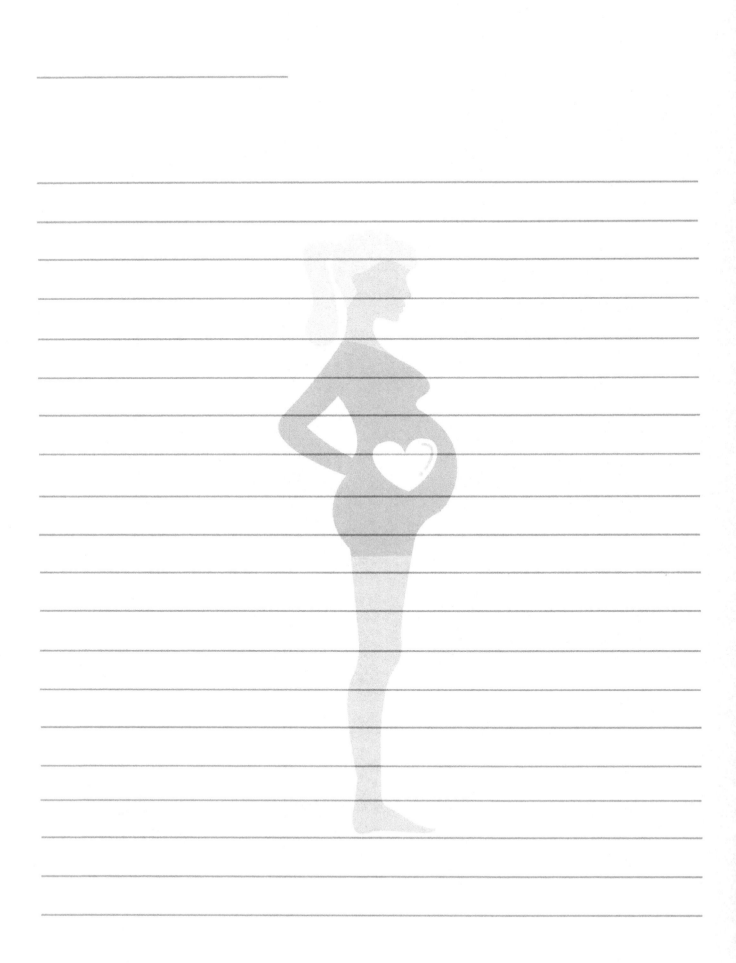

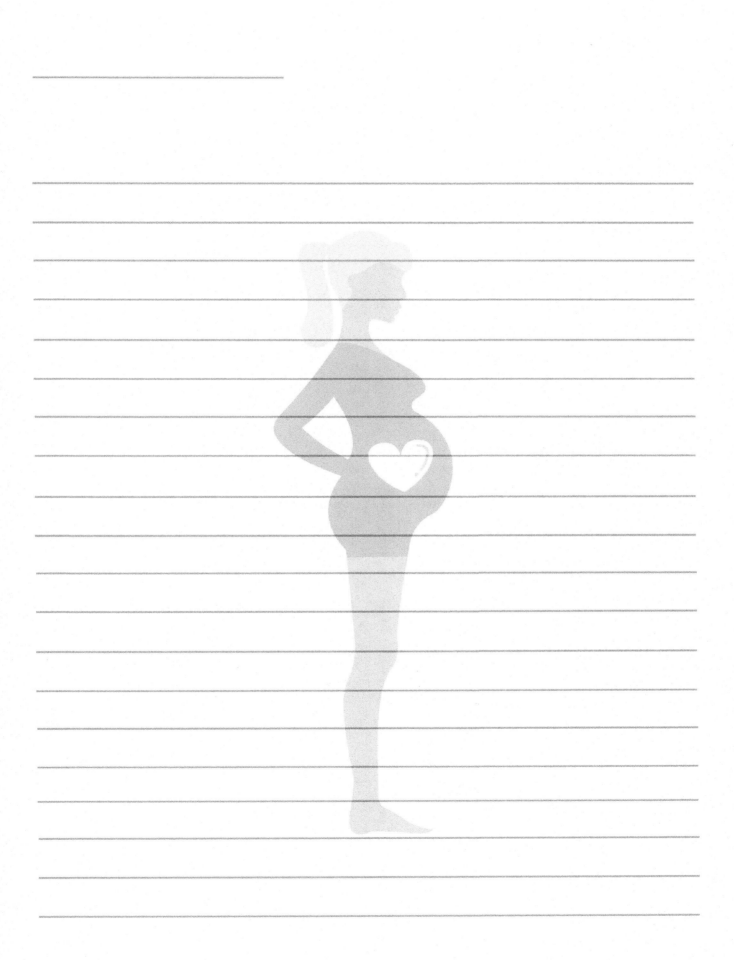

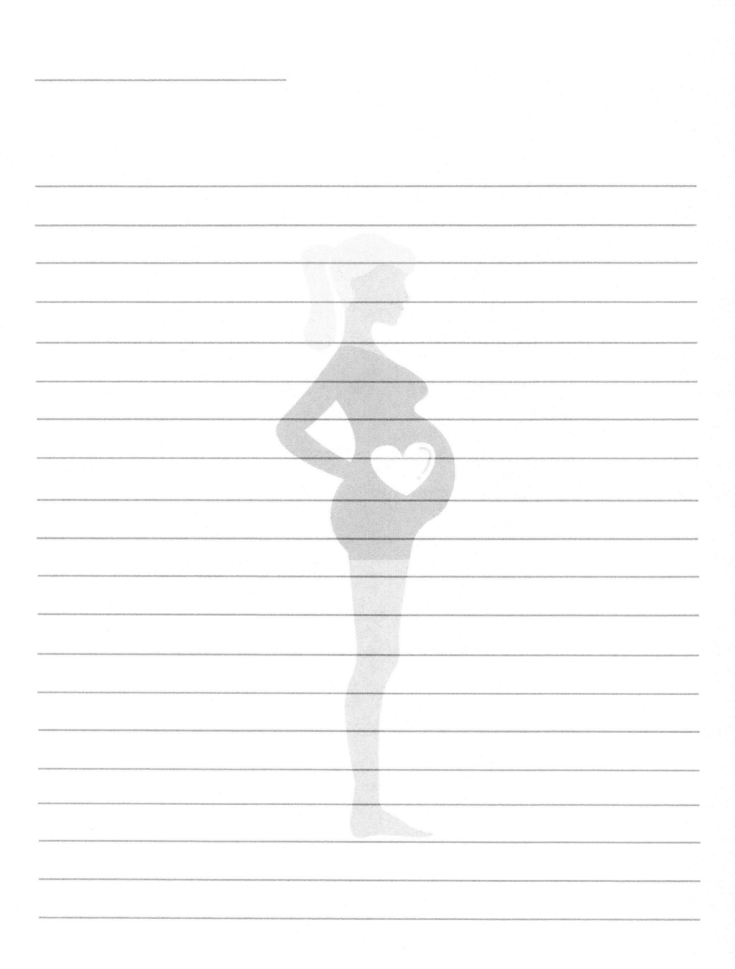

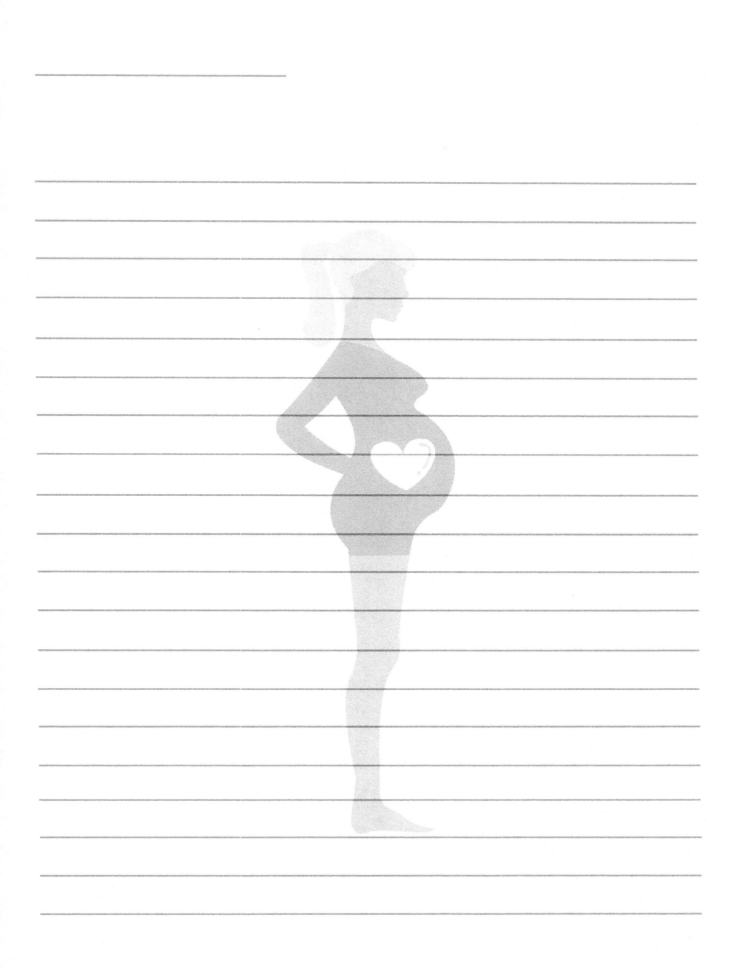

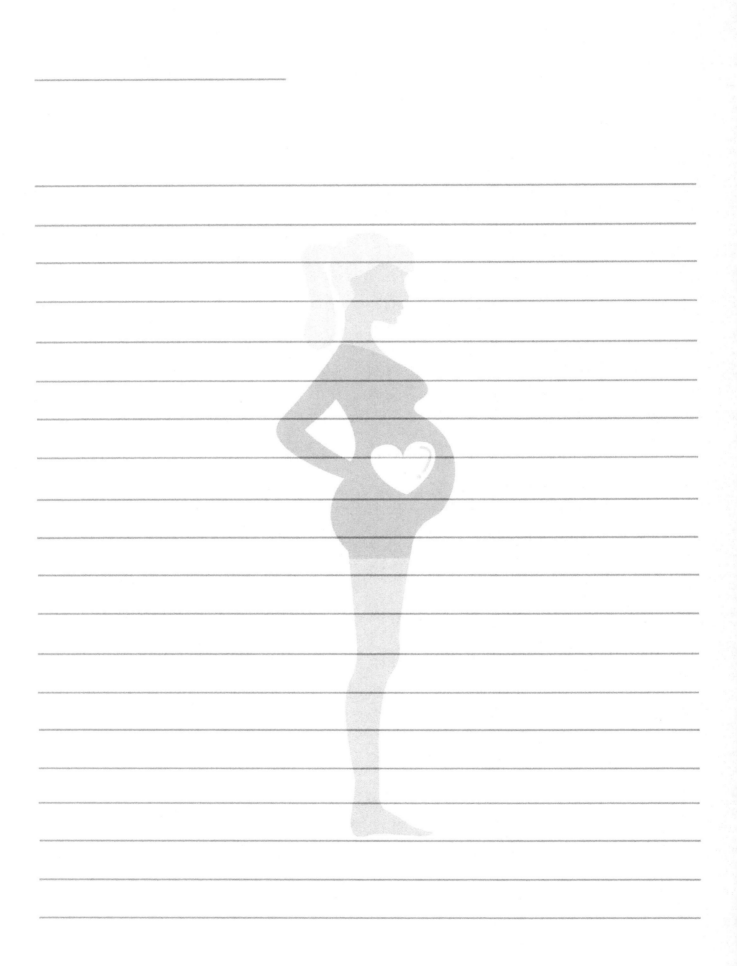

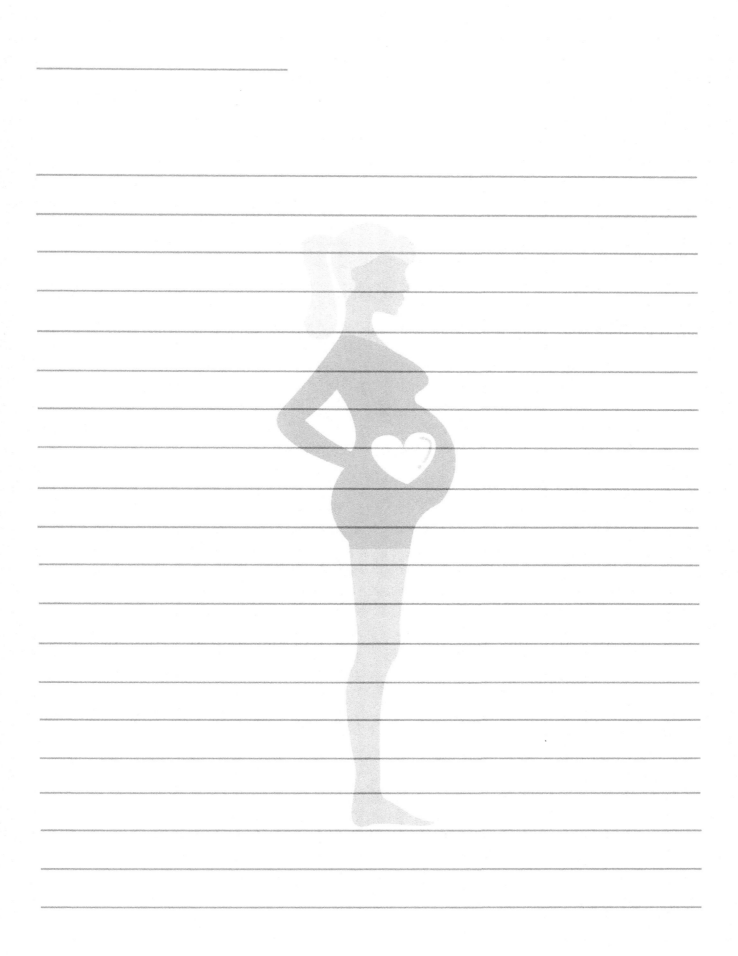

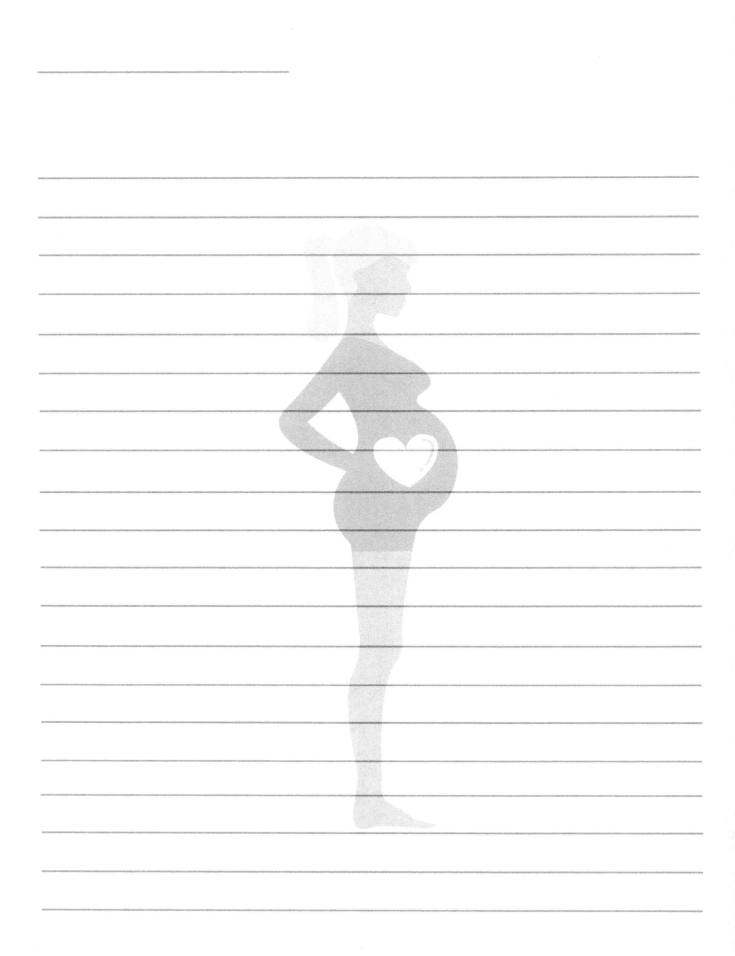

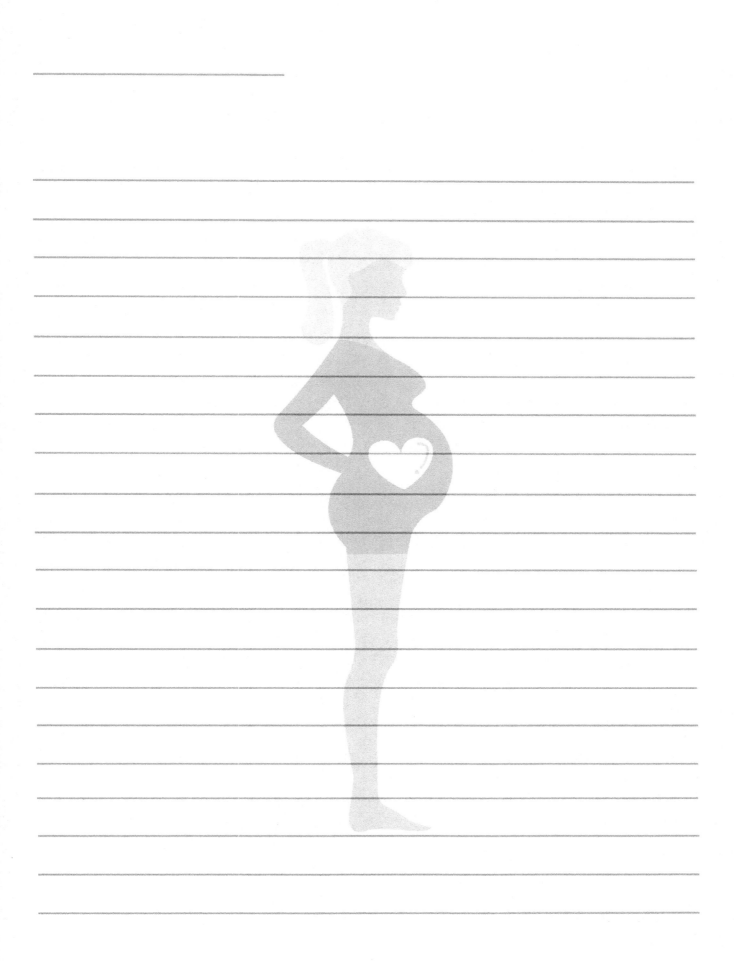

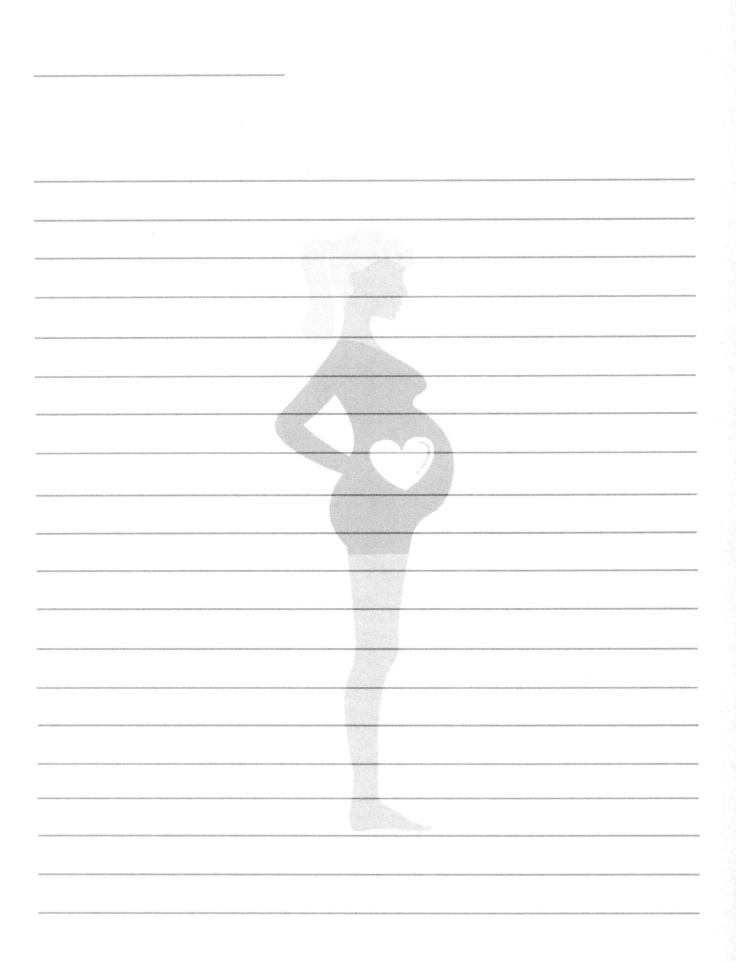

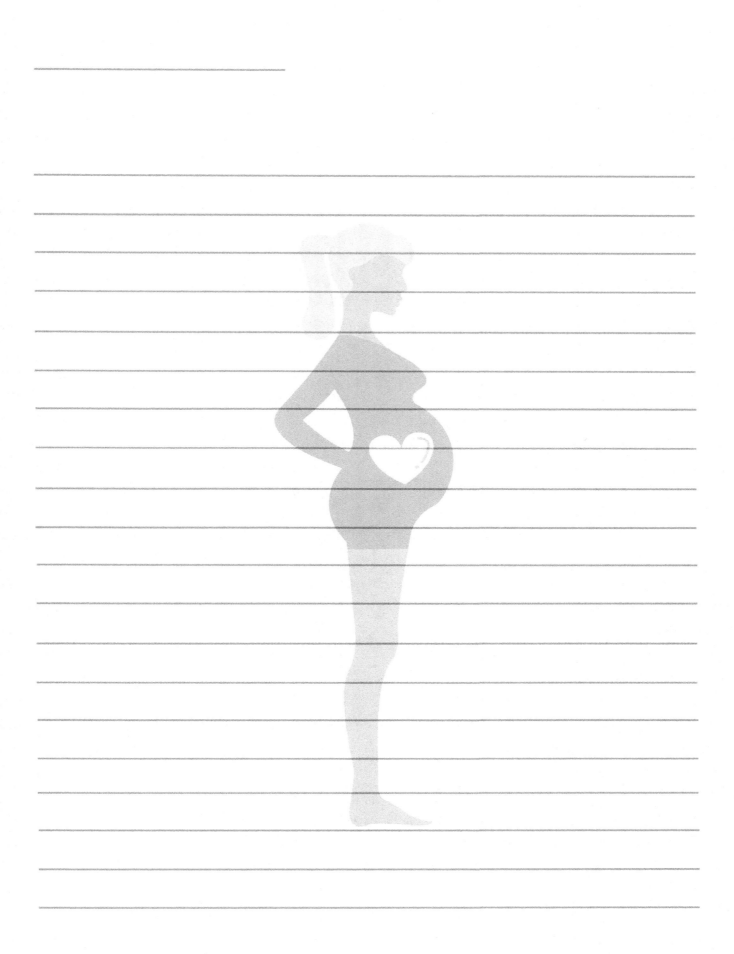

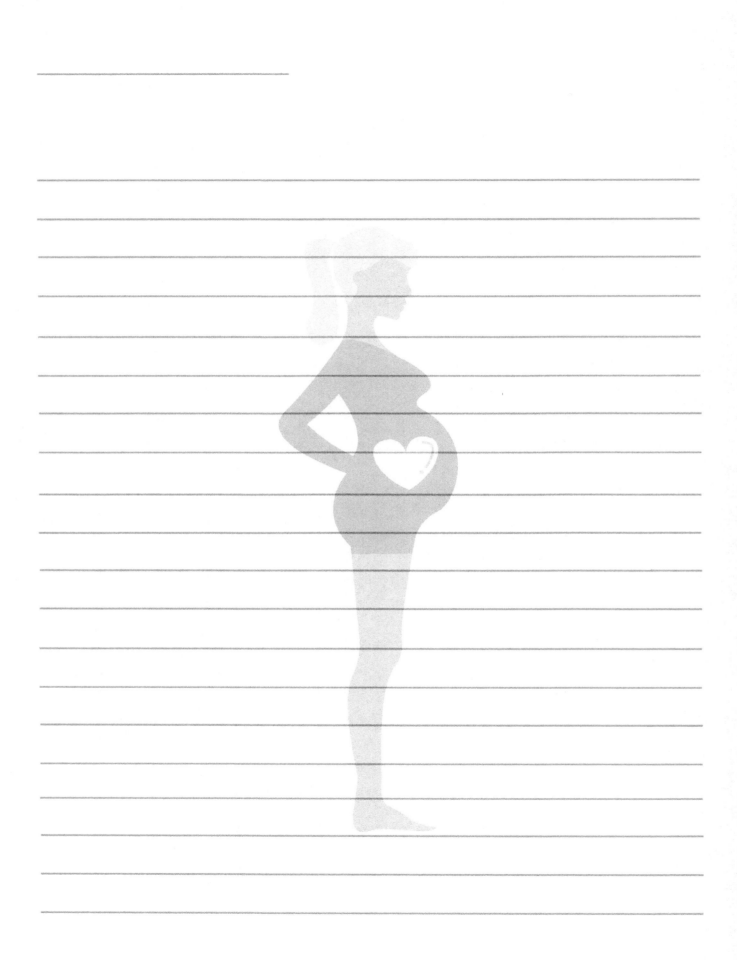

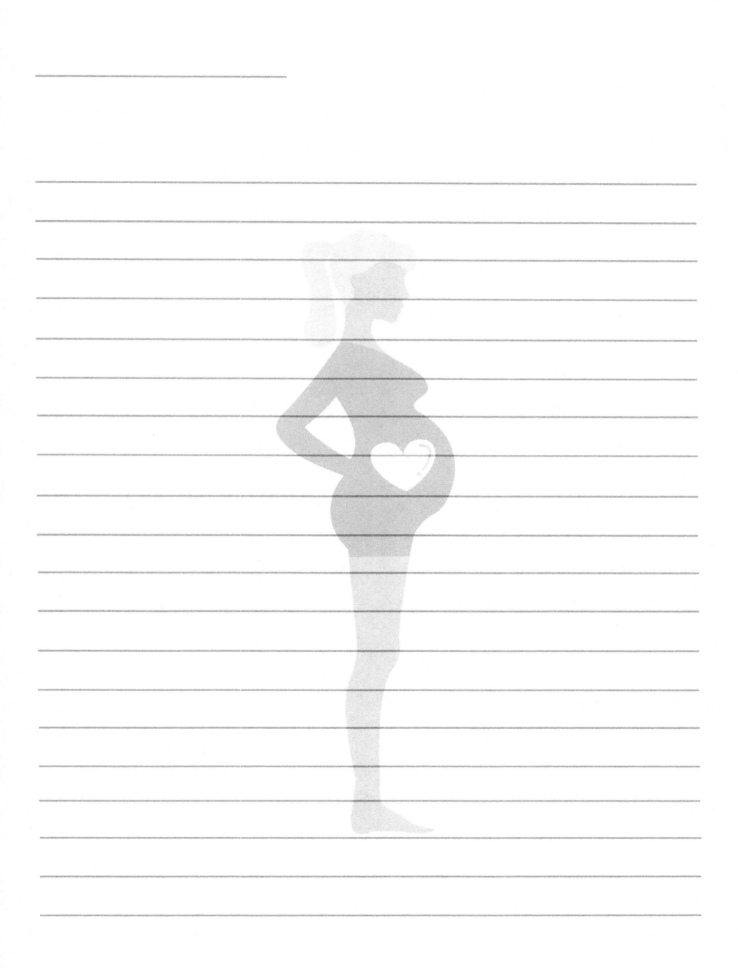

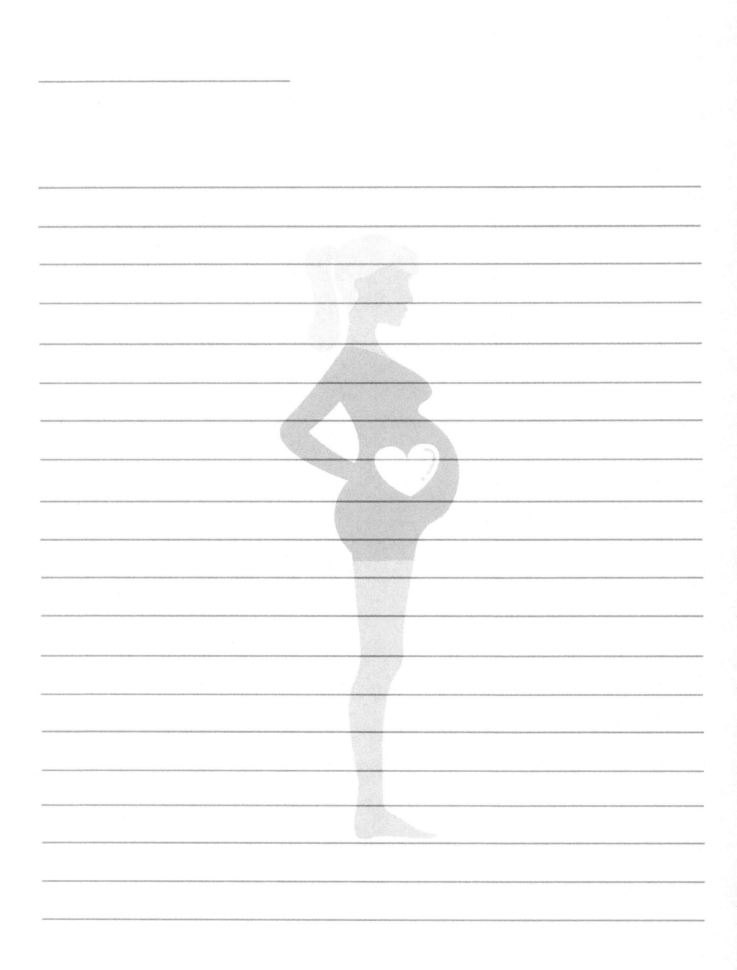

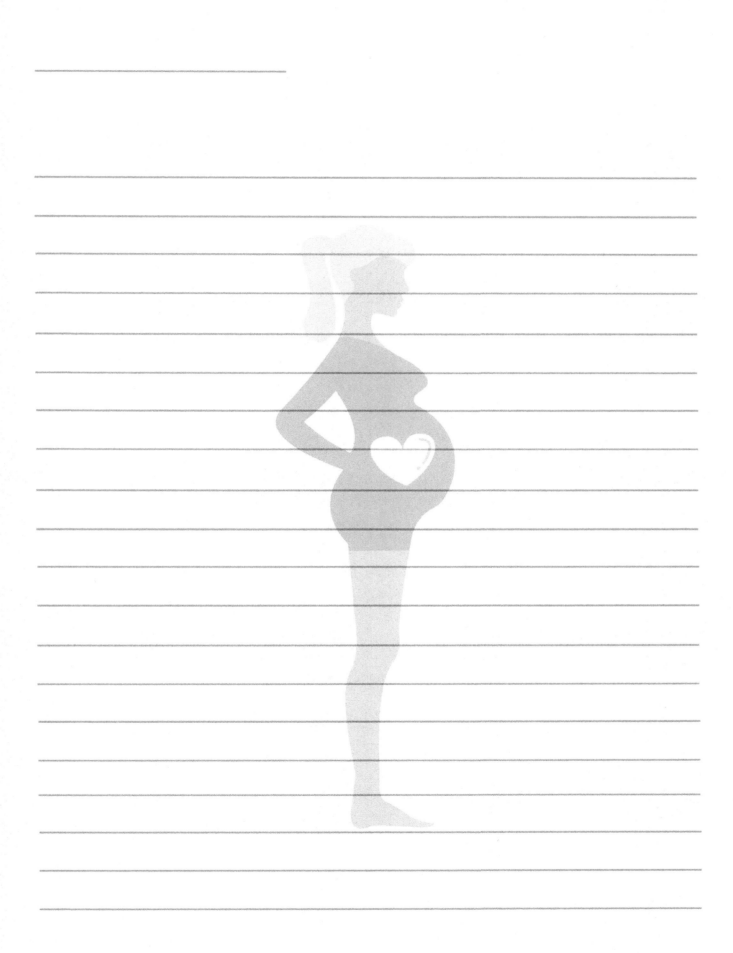

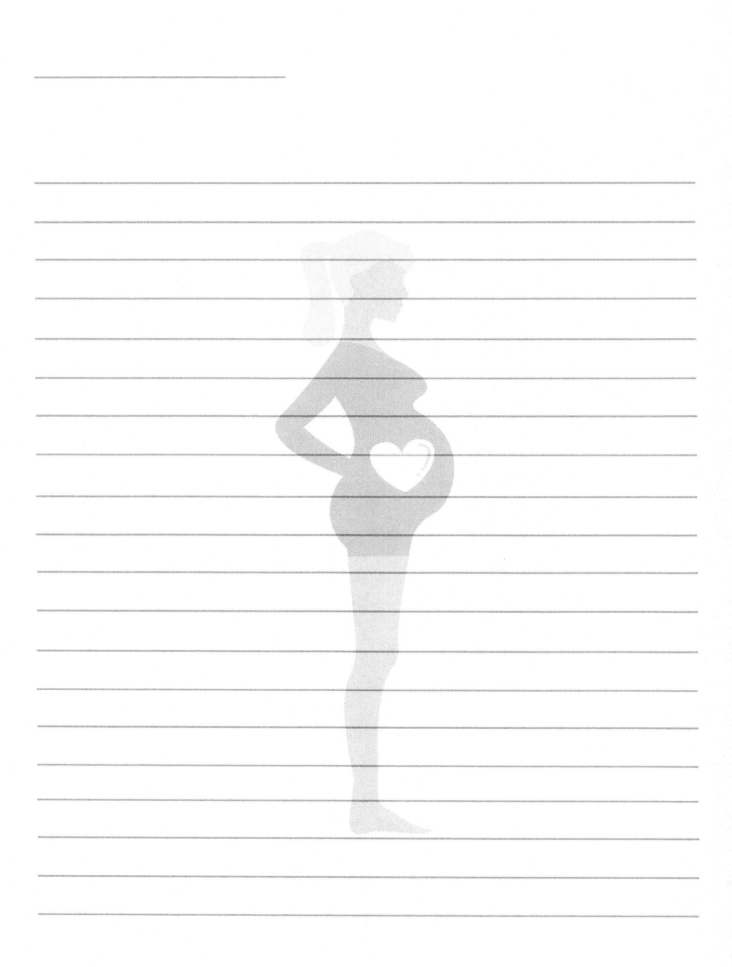

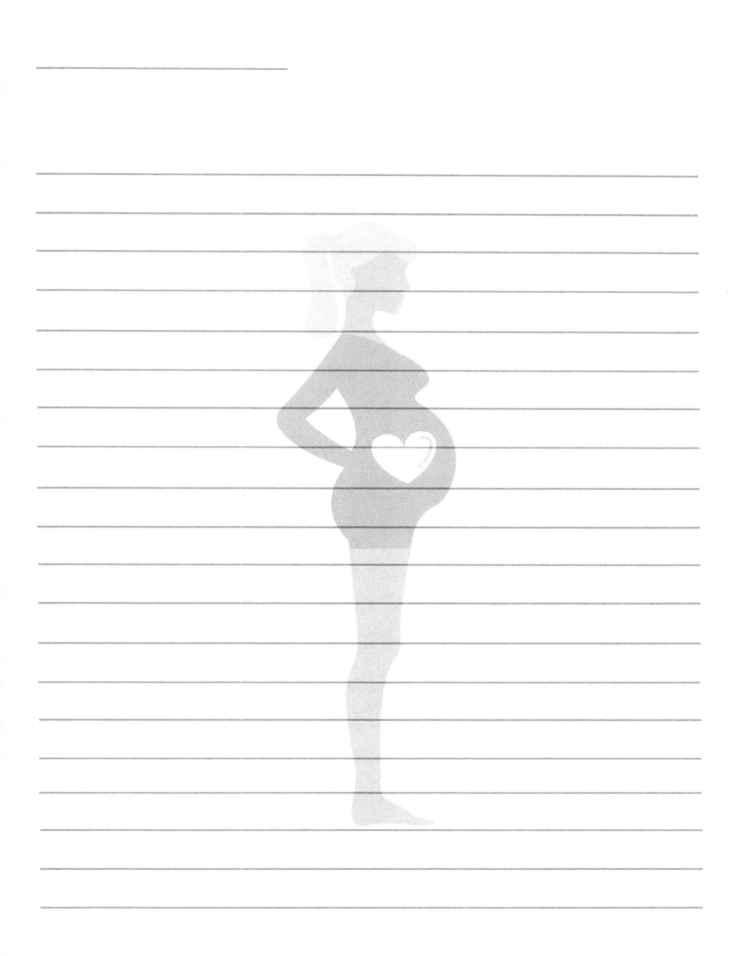

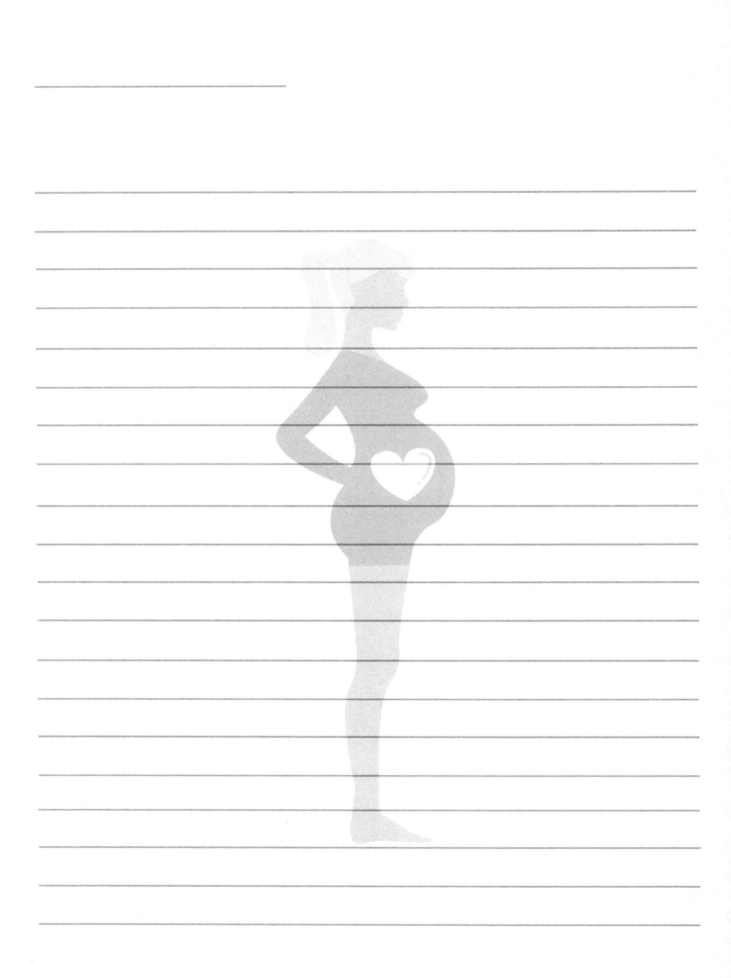

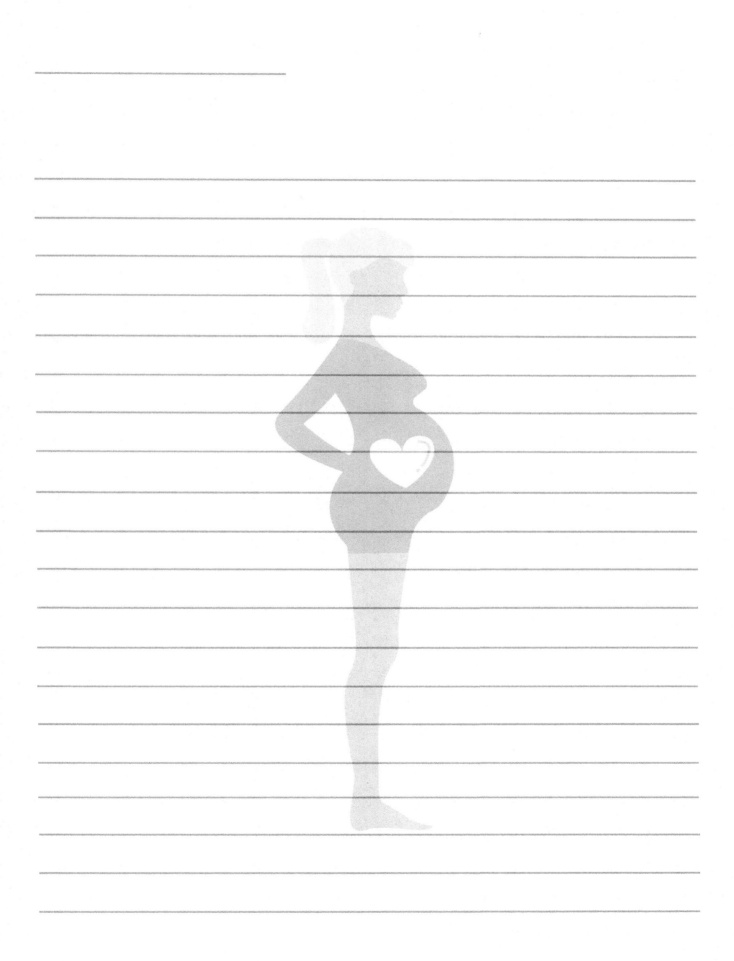

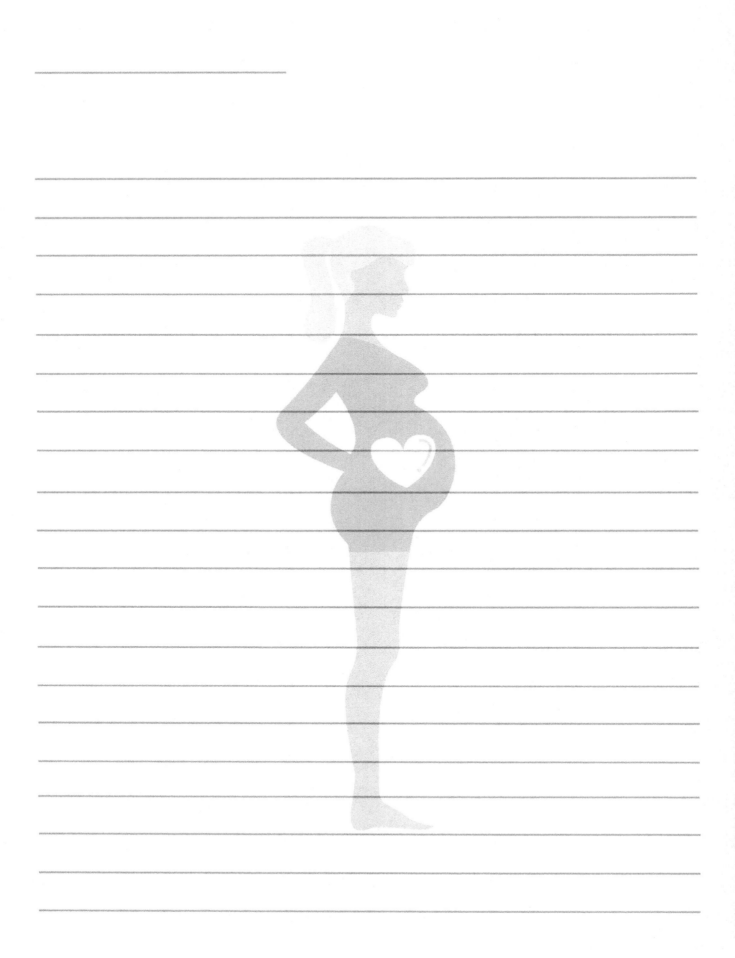

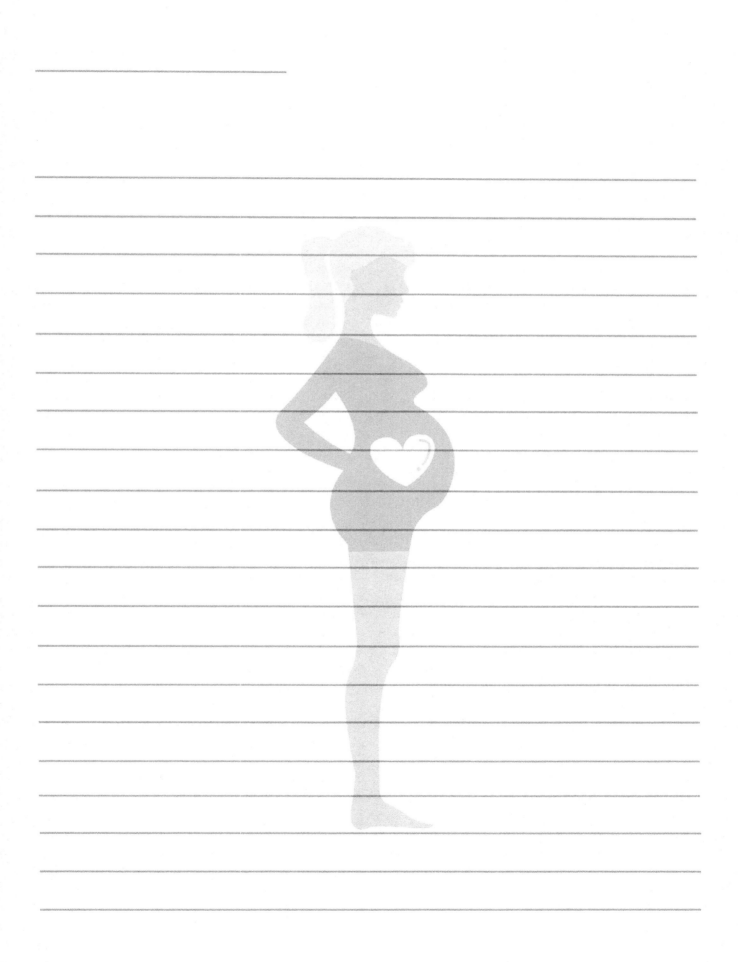

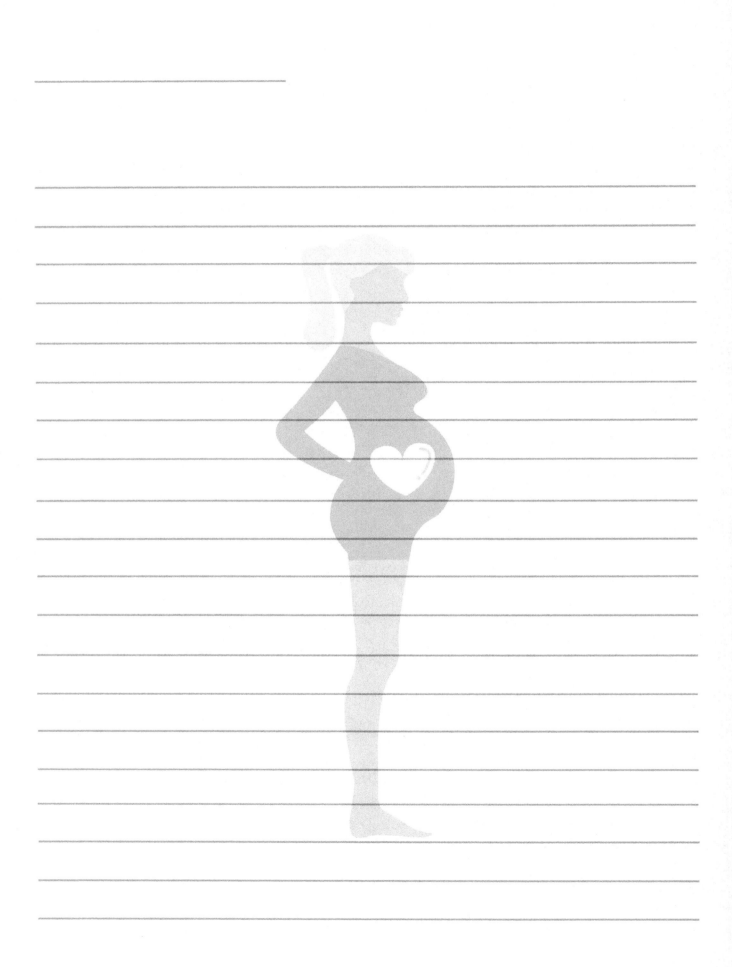

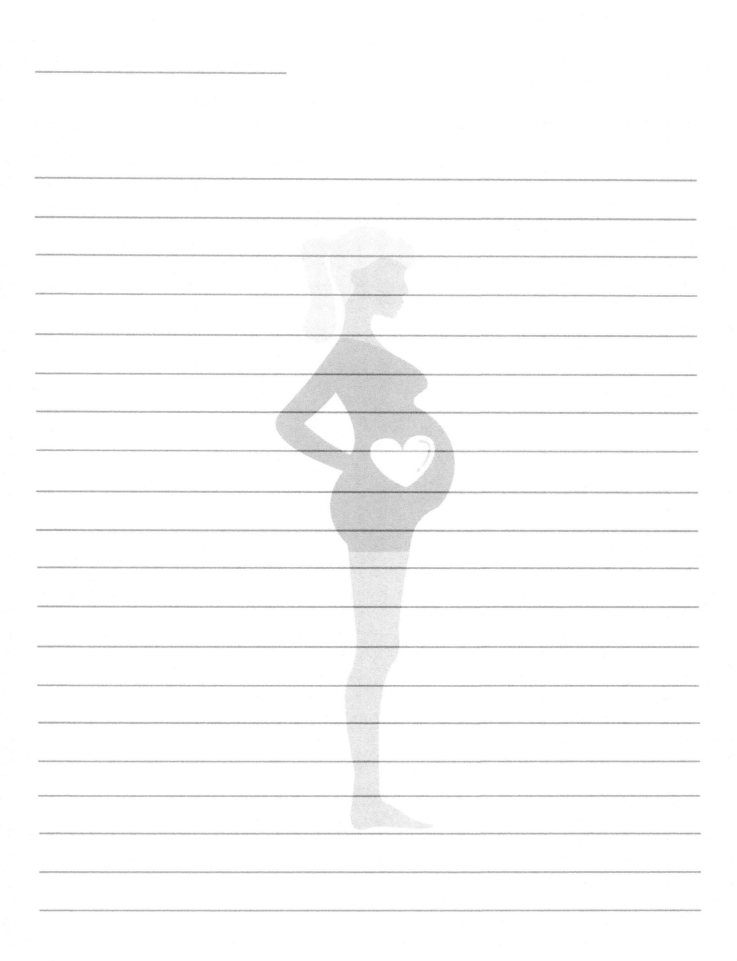

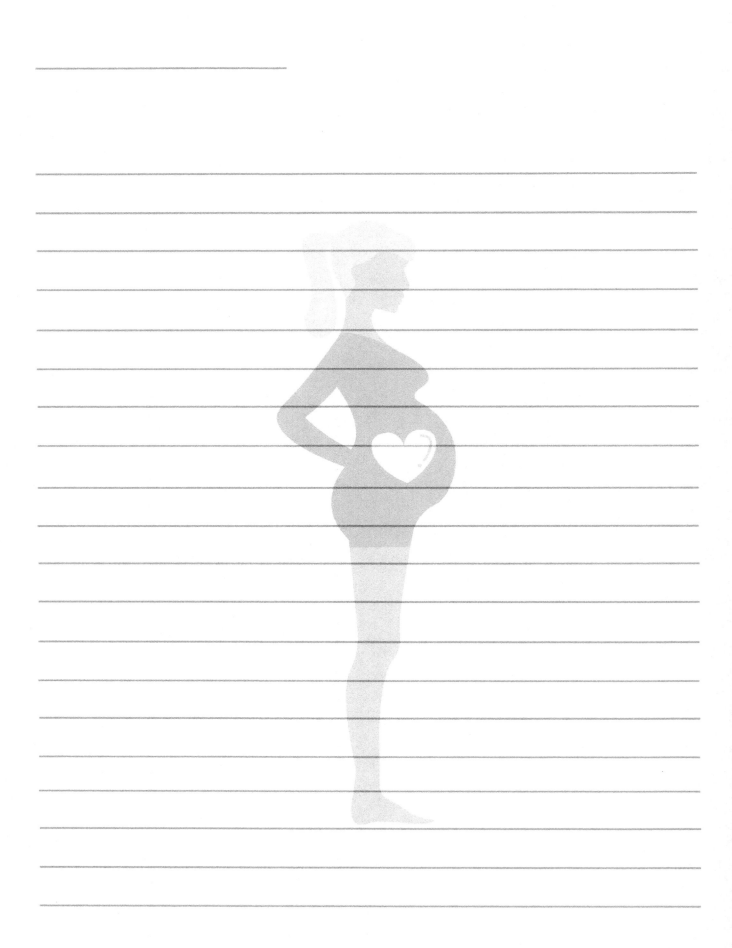

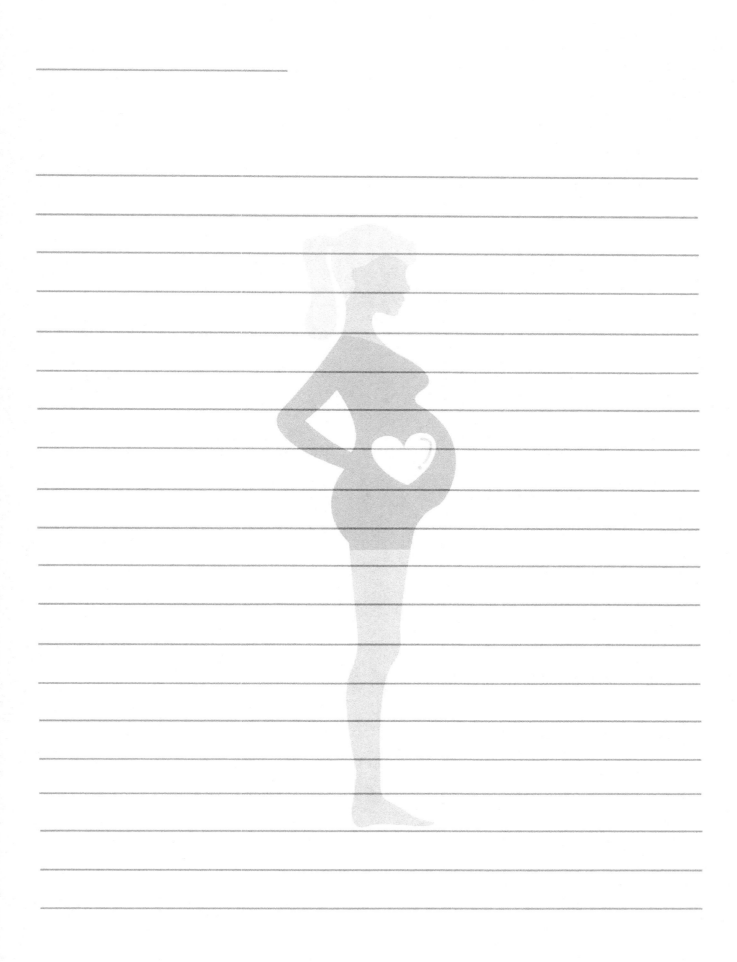

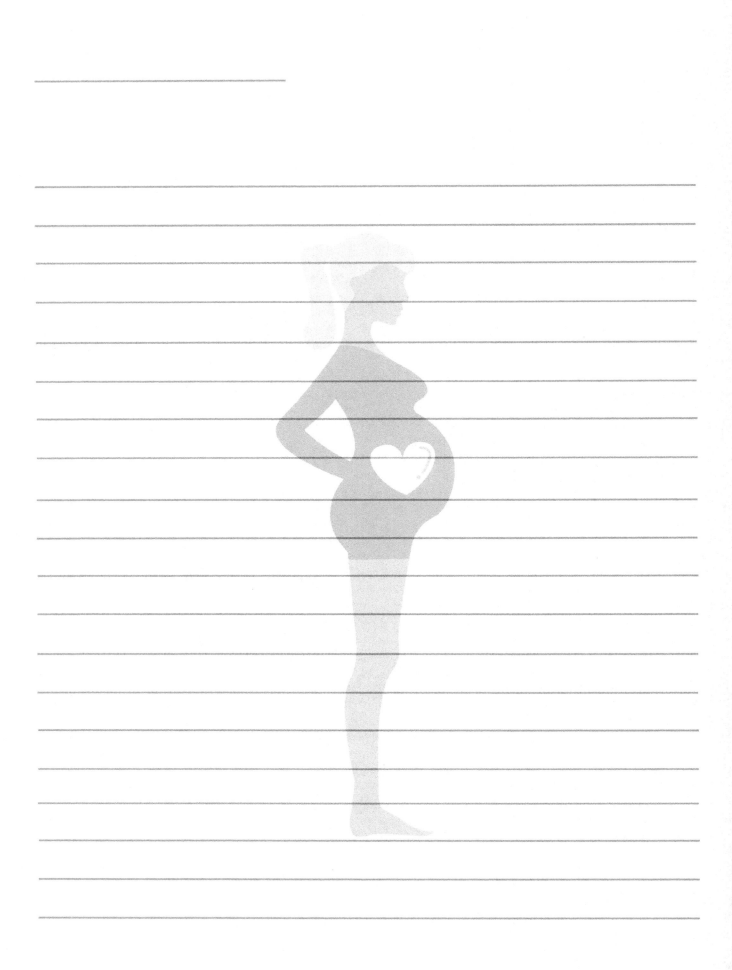

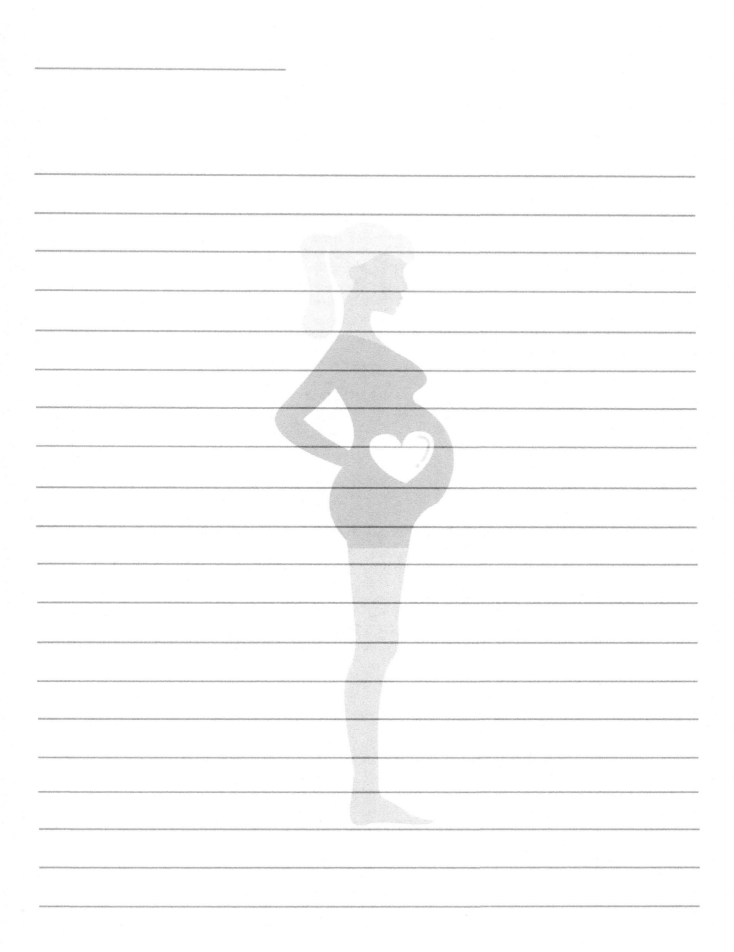

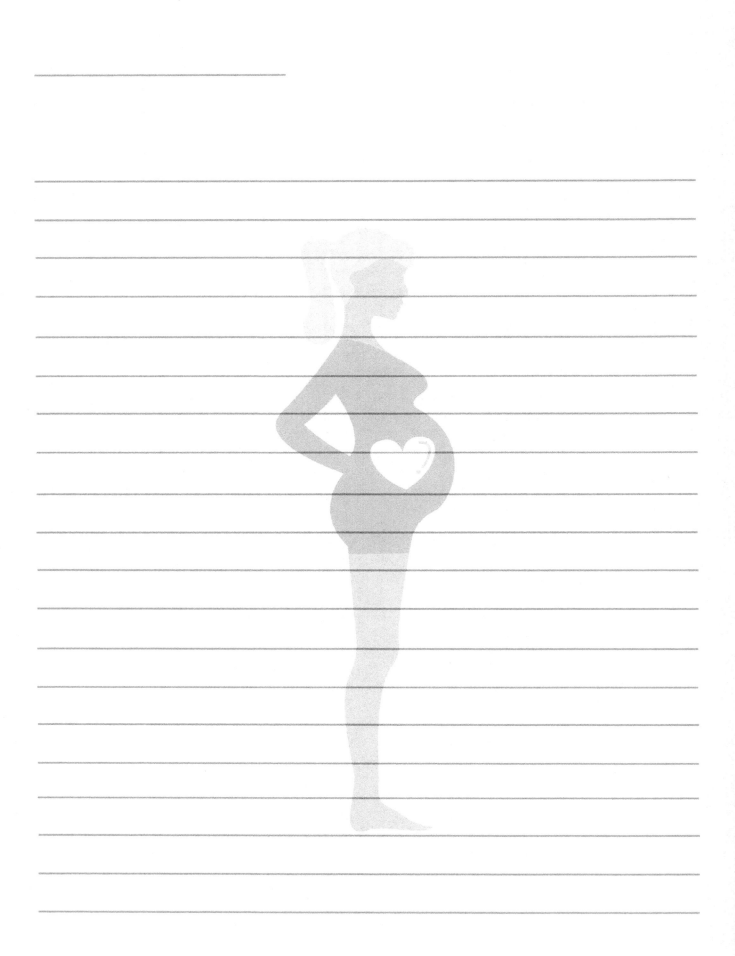

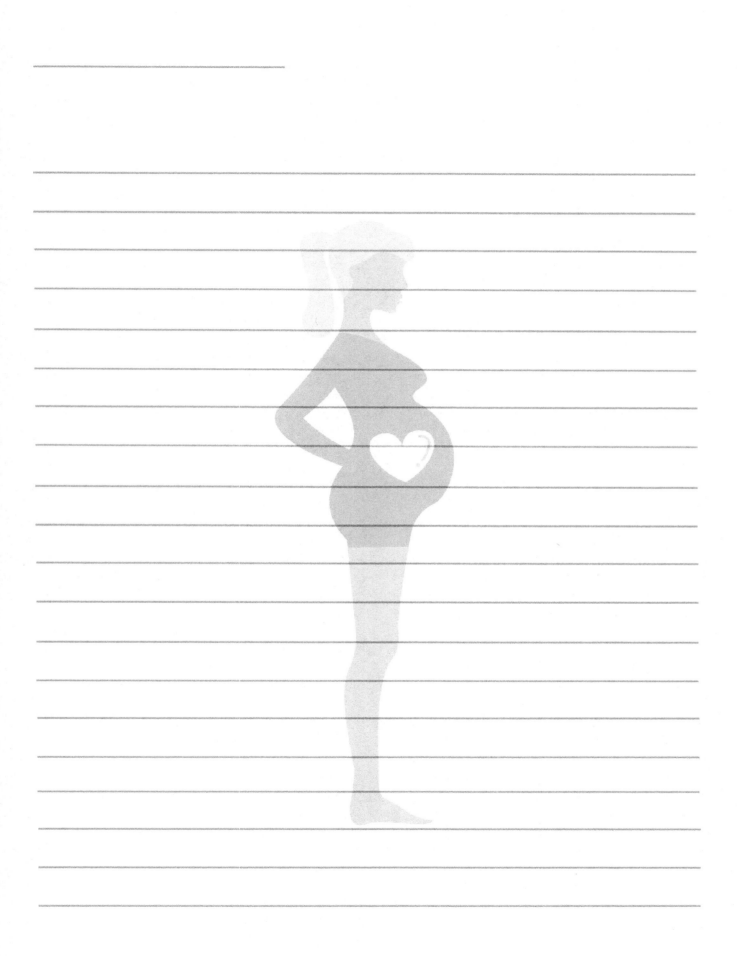

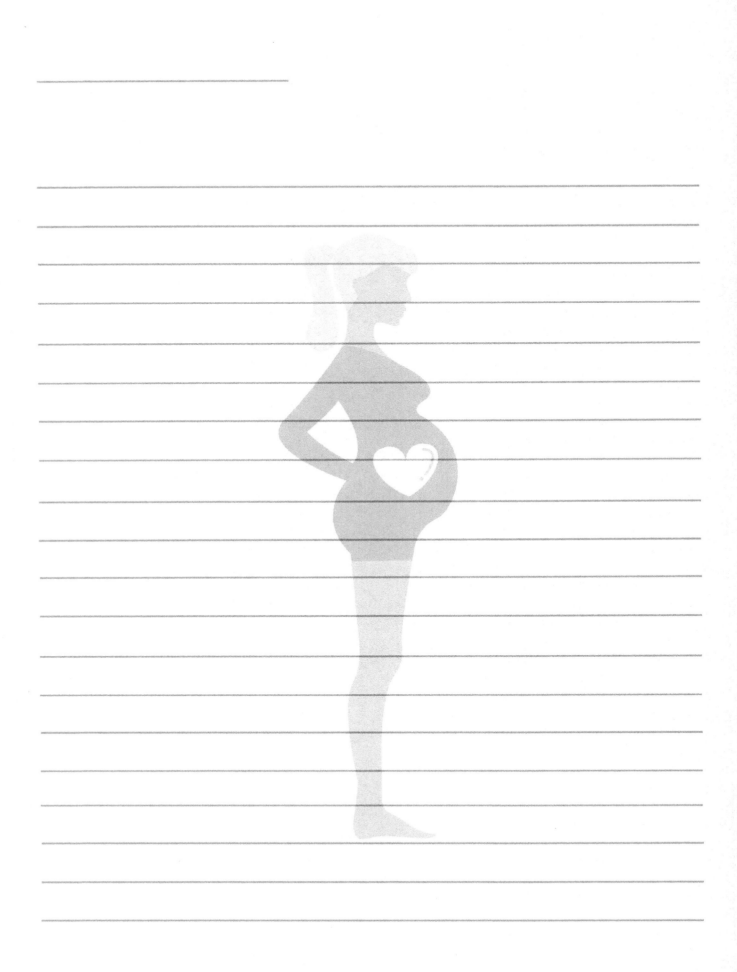

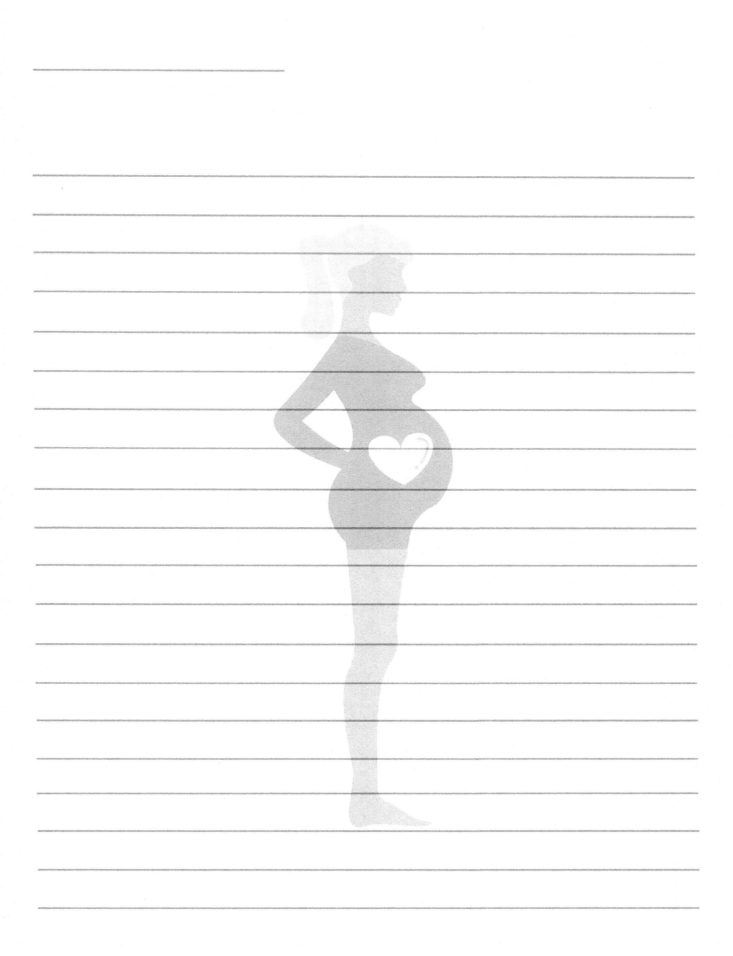

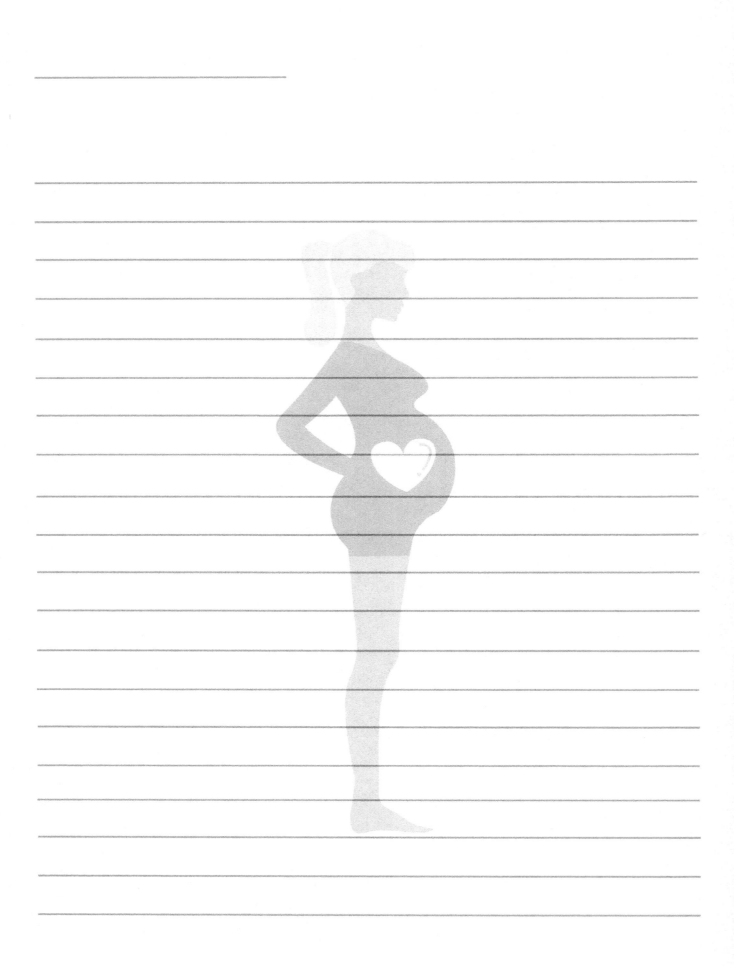

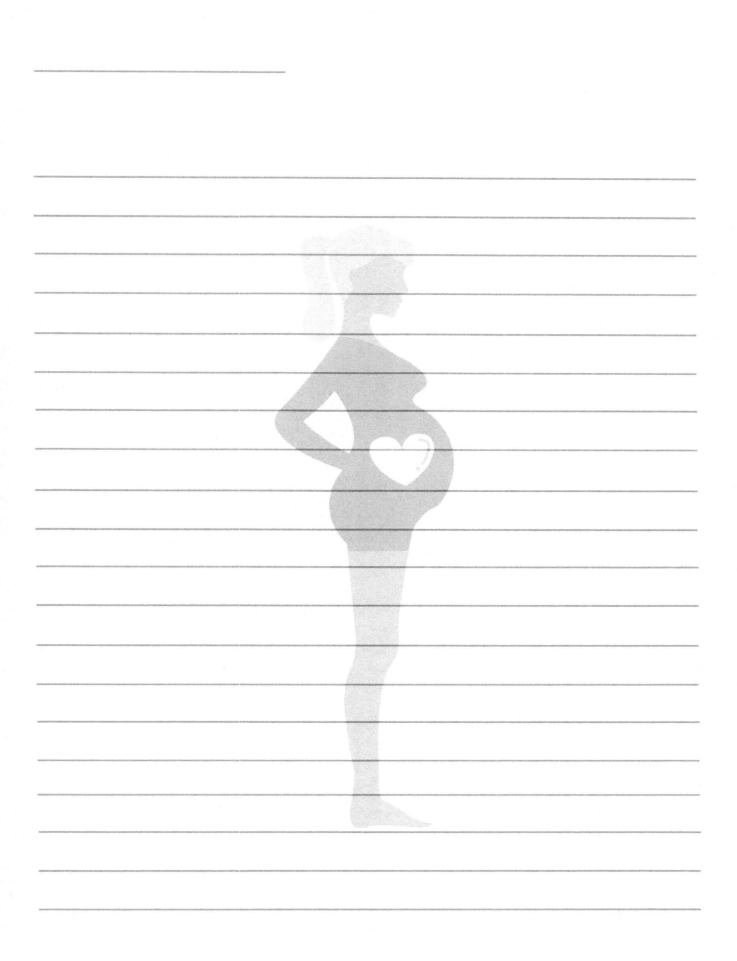

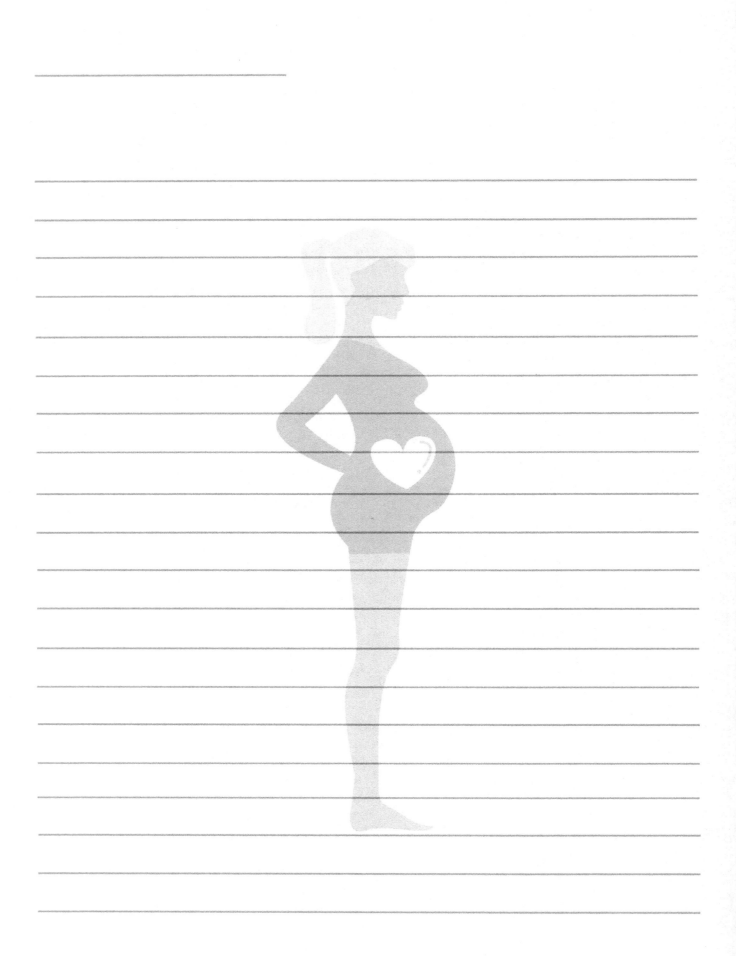

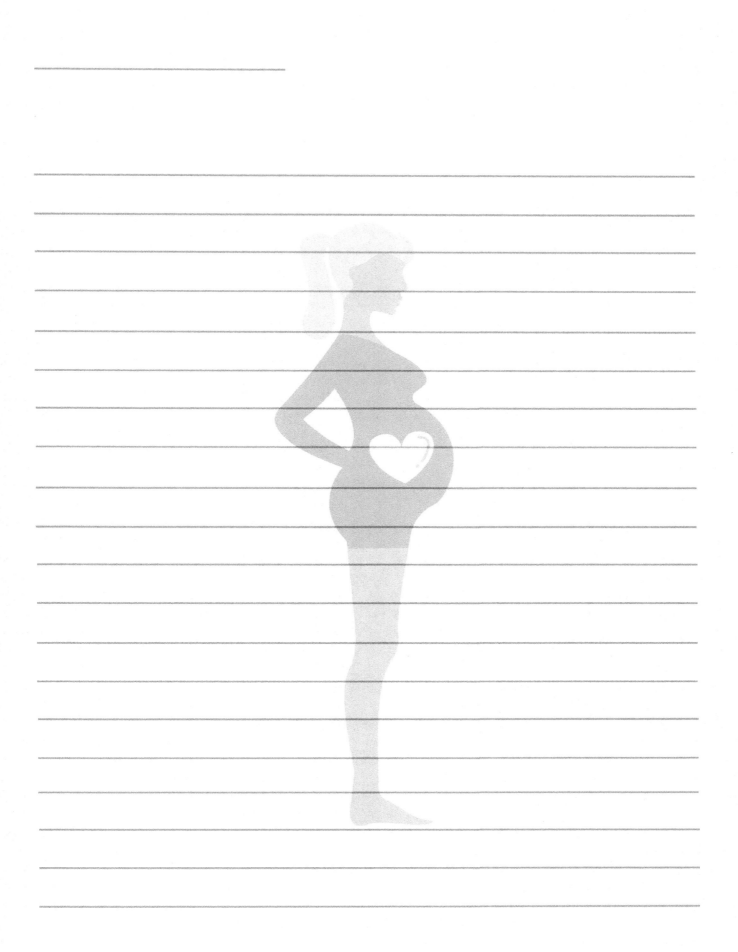

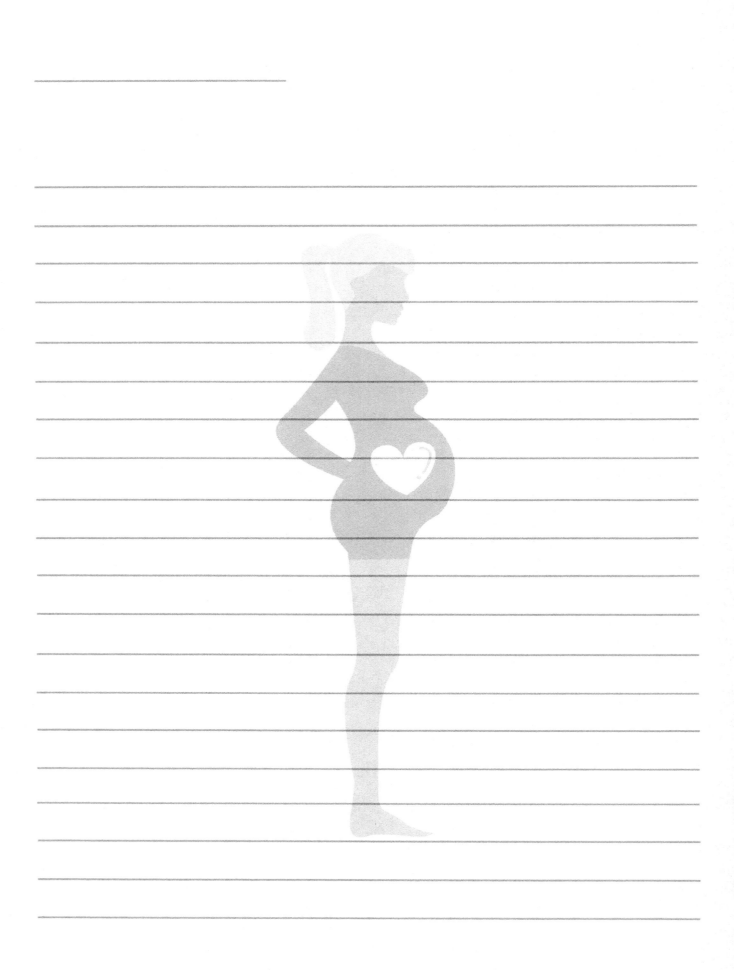

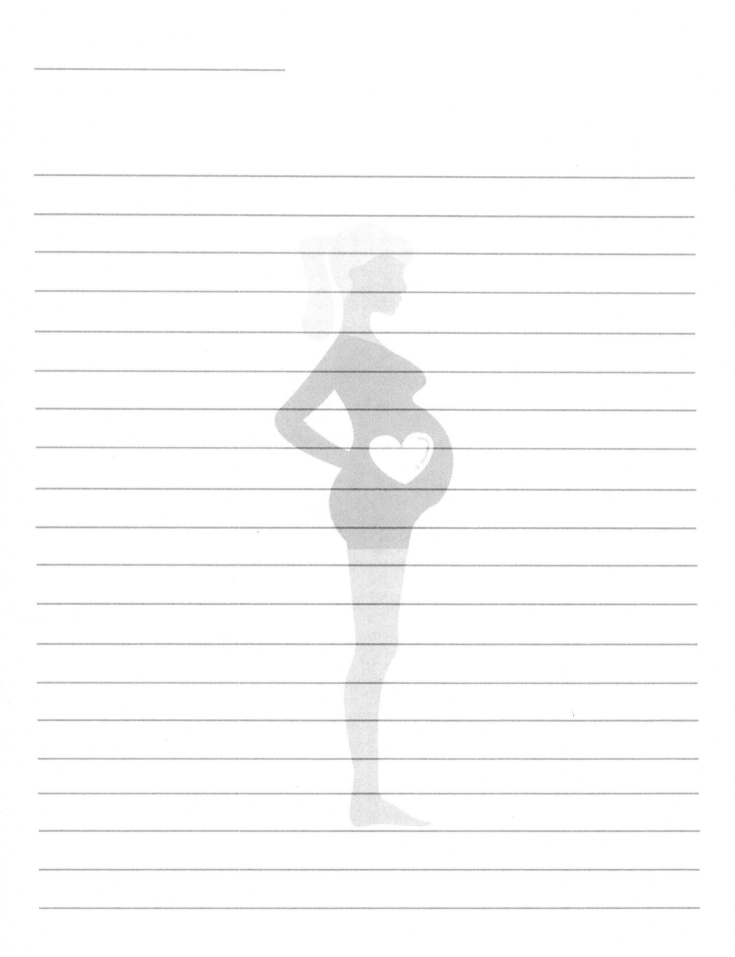

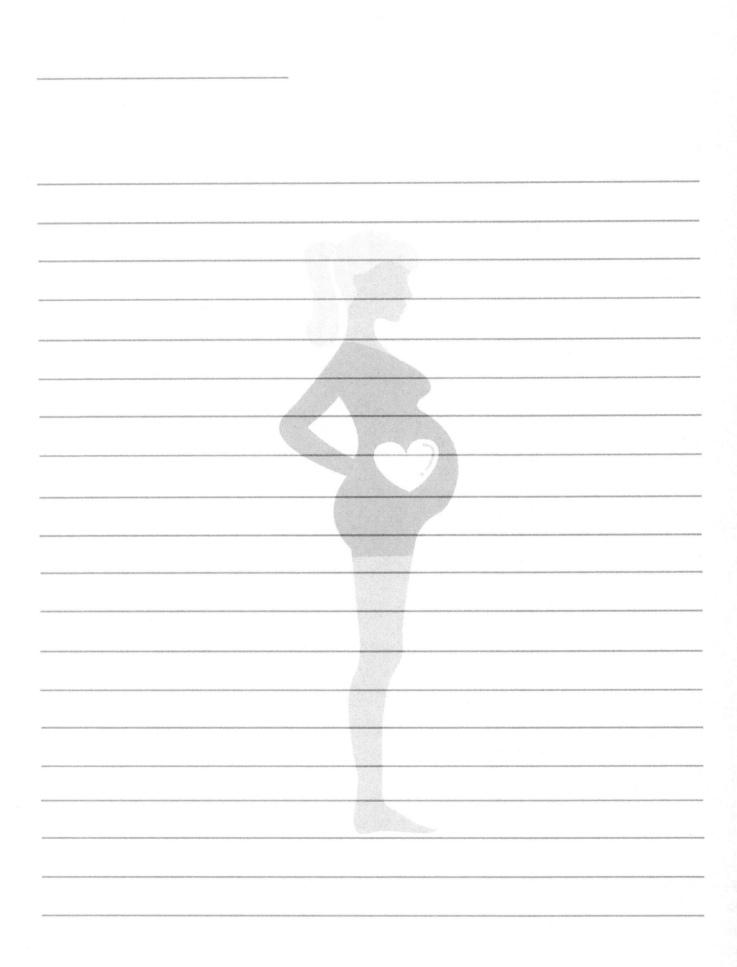

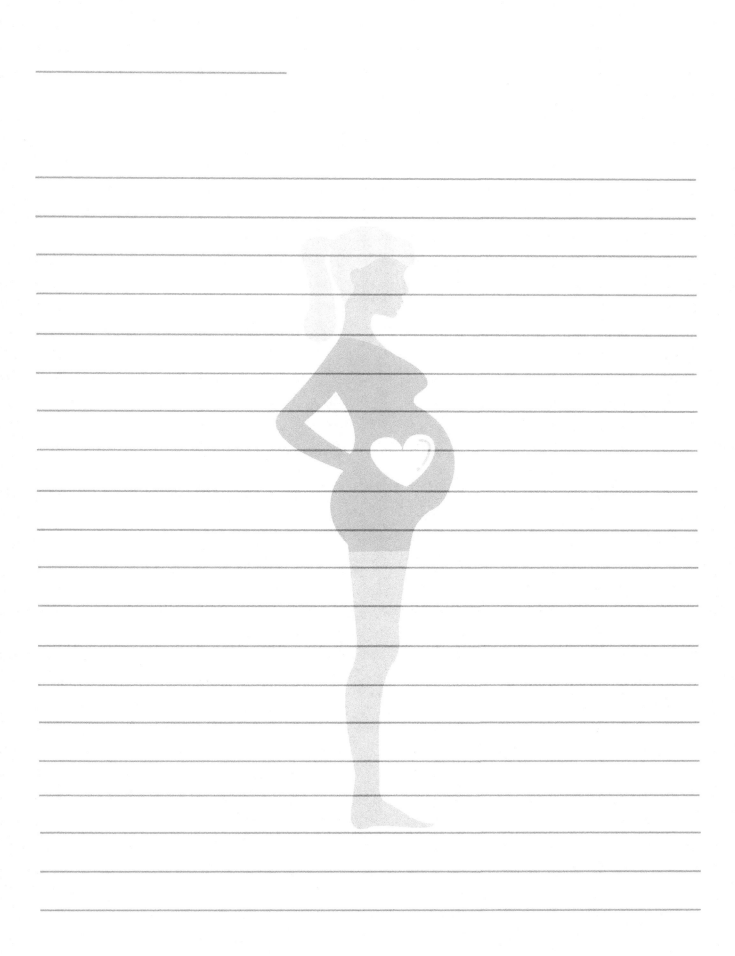

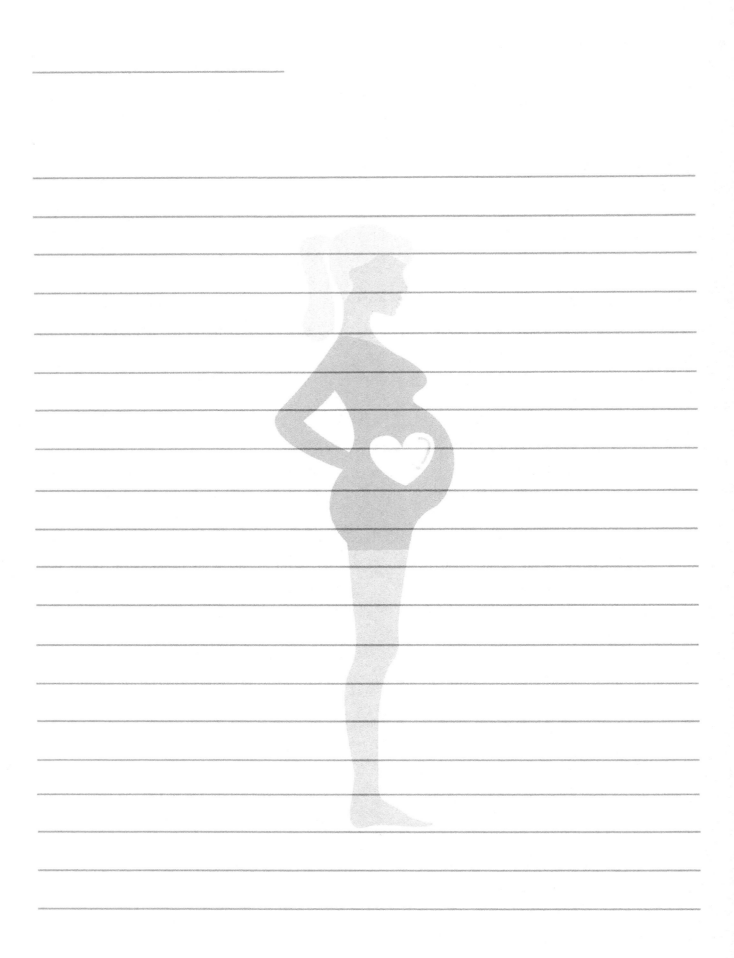

Made in United States
North Haven, CT
22 June 2022

20498734R00111